Dedication
For Lynn and Boz, who helped more than they know

For Elsevier:

Publisher: Steven Black
Development Editor: Katrina Mather/Gill Cloke
Project Manager: Joannah Duncan
Design: Erik Bigland
Illustrator: Jane Fallows

Neuropsychology
for Nurses and Allied Health Professionals

Chris Green C Psychol
Neuropsychologist

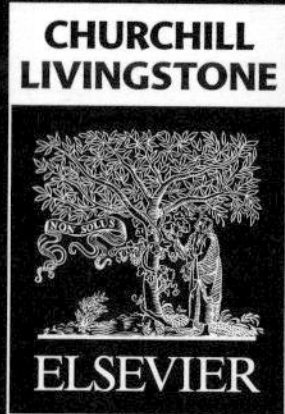

EDINBURGH LONDON NEW YORK OXFORD PHILADELPHIA
ST LOUIS SYDNEY TORONTO 2006

CHURCHILL
LIVINGSTONE
ELSEVIER

First published 2006

ISBN 0 443 10106 X

British Library Cataloguing in Publication Data
A catalogue record for this book is available from the British Library

Library of Congress Cataloging in Publication Data
A catalog record for this book is available from the Library of Congress

Notice
Medical knowledge is constantly changing. Standard safety precautions must be followed, but as new research and clinical experience broaden our knowledge, changes in treatment and drug therapy may become necessary or appropriate. Readers are advised to check the most current product information provided by the manufacturer of each drug to be administered to verify the recommended dose, the method and duration of administration, and contraindications. It is the responsibility of the practitioner, relying on experience and knowledge of the patient, to determine dosages and the best treatment for each individual patient. Neither the Publisher nor the author assumes any liability for any injury and/or damage to persons or property arising from this publication.
The Publisher

The publisher's policy is to use paper manufactured from sustainable forests

Printed in China

PREFACE

It was while lecturing to qualified and pre-registration nurses that I first became aware that there was no specific text available that concisely mapped the intricacies of neuropsychology; there was no reference material that clearly defined the subject without going into too much detail; and there was no detailed resource available to members of a care team responsible for ministering to the needs of specific patients for many more hours in the day than I.

I also became aware that the brain, with all its complex functions and subtle (and sometimes not so subtle) influences on behaviour, tended to be viewed either as just another organ of the body to be treated in much the same way as a liver or a spleen, or as a mysterious and forbidding territory that produced individual action by some curious and almost inexplicable process.

Of course neither of these two somewhat extreme positions is correct. The brain and neuropsychological performance are neither as mundane as simple homeostatic functioning nor as alarming as the production of behaviour from the unknown. Instead, the truth lies somewhere in the middle ground which constantly changes as our greater understanding pushes back the veils of our ignorance.

A useful example would be the case of epilepsy. In ancient times the condition was often seen as demon possession. Our understanding grew but we could still not exactly define the condition and so it became known largely as what it appeared to be, 'falling down sickness'. More recently, and as a result of our greater medical sophistication, we have come to refer to the condition as epilepsy. No longer attributing the electrophysiological disturbances of the brain to possession, we address the disorder as a medical entity, governed by physiological processes and amenable, as is often the case, to medications that can return the sufferer to a normal life.

Over and above these historical changes in nomenclature, however, what is of particular interest to the neuropsychologist is that so often the behaviour which can be associated with epilepsy can be misunderstood or misinterpreted as signs of another, usually psychological or psychiatric condition. For example: gelastic seizures involve involuntary laughing, while dacrystic seizures involve involuntary crying; temporal lobe epilepsy can produce complex visual hallucinations, while ecstatic epilepsy can produce feelings of harmony and a god-like relationship with the world.

Conversely, it is not unusual for patients with psychological or psychiatric difficulties to experience non-epileptic seizures that can be mistaken for electrographic seizures and, thus, be steered into investigations and medication trials that were probably unnecessary.

In both of these cases, then, an understanding of the brain, its workings, and neuropsychology can help to transform a complex presentation into something more accessible. A presentation that on the surface might appear bizarre can then be turned into something that we are able to assess, investigate, and treat. This does not mean that there are no more mysterious and fascinating boundaries to cross in our endeavour to understand the complexities of medical neuroscience, because there are: for every question answered, there seem to be ten more questions to ask. Little by little we come to comprehend more, seeing things in a new light, transmitting this new knowledge to patients and, thus, providing them with a greater understanding of what can often be tremendously traumatic conditions accompanied by equally dramatic life changes.

On first being ushered into the field of neuropsychology, I was naive enough to believe that the brain and its chemical, electrophysiological and anatomical components could offer a complex circuit diagram to aid in my understanding of behaviour, emotion, cognition and perception. I was soon to learn, however, that these physiological mechanisms were only the beginning of a long and meandering path that, despite their highly structured nature, could not at that time fully encapsulate the sum of human experience.

To illustrate simply: if we have a headache, we take aspirin and the pain goes away; however, it was not a lack of aspirin that caused the headache in the first place. And so it is with neuropsychology. What you see is not necessarily what you get!

In teaching these principles, I have often amused students by asking them to think of themselves as patients being told their diagnosis for the first time. Invariably, I have used the example of a patient being told that they have epistaxis or post-prandial upper abdominal distension. At first glance, these labels would appear to have a worryingly medical quality that might have you or me reaching for a medical dictionary or worse. However, when it is explained that epistaxis is a nose bleed and post-prandial upper abdominal distension is a bloating of the abdomen caused by the accumulation of gas after eating dinner, the fear that one might have something serious tends to evaporate.

Similarly, patients experiencing dysmnesia after a head injury or dysgeusia after a stroke might be so overpowered by the jargon that it becomes very difficult to reach the person to whom these symptoms are attached. It is only when dysmnesia and dysgeusia are expressed as poor memory and a dysfunction of the sense of taste that these symptoms can be put in their correct perspective as a function of the patient's illness or trauma.

Part of the purpose of this book, therefore, is to increase the reader's knowledge and confidence with reference to some of the common and not so common neuropsychological symptoms and presentations associated with neurological illness and trauma and, thereby, provide an insight into what is truly an absorbing and intriguing discipline. The other purpose of this text, however, is to offer the reader a resource from which to expand their own understanding and, hopefully, pass this understanding on to other practitioners and, more importantly, patients.

To this end we will, in the first part of this text, take a brief tour of the history of neuropsychology, introduce or re-acquaint ourselves with basic neuroanatomy and functional neuroanatomy, look at the different types of neuroradiological and neuroimaging techniques currently used, and consider the medical and neuropsychological symptoms and presentations of some of the more common conditions. In the second part of the text we will apply ourselves to some of the less well-known disorders, address the issue of neuropsychological assessment, and look at the mechanisms of recovery and rehabilitation. Finally, we will make a foray into some of the more common pharmacological interventions used and provide a guide to additional resources such as websites, journals and disorder-specific support groups.

Where possible I have used positional terminology to denote the placement of sites within the brain and explanations of neuropsychological and neurological terms. This has been done so as not to burden the reader with an off-putting feat that would test the skills of a linguist, but in order to provide an introduction to the array of language used within this discipline. This, of course, is supported by a glossary of terms, which can be found in the appendices. However, in the spirit of the old saying 'those who cry at funerals should not become undertakers', I believe that some exposure to these terms is an inevitable consequence of enquiring into the field of neuroscience.

Nevertheless, I am also mindful that some of the texts available for undergraduate and postgraduate neuropsychological study can be somewhat daunting in terms of their depth and prodigious length. Here, then, it was my intent to create a store of information that was more accessible to those that required only the essential elements necessary for understanding and, more importantly, the provision of care. Should the reader, however, wish to enquire further in more detail, I have taken the liberty of presenting a further reading list at the end of each chapter.

To conclude, then, it is my hope that those reading this text will develop a new understanding and respect for the neurological conditions of their patients, which is garnered from a specialty that offers a different perspective and seeks to synthesize a view of symptoms with the person that presents in a truly holistic manner.

Chris Green
July 2005

CONTENTS

What is neuropsychology?

1

OVERVIEW

I am often asked: 'What is neuropsychology?' To which my reply, just as often, is that in its strictest sense:

> Neuropsychology is the study of the relationship between brain structure and behaviour that seeks to understand how behaviour, emotion, cognition, and perception may be related to and underpinned by the chemical, electrophysiological, anatomical and integrative processes of the central nervous system with the broad aim of the assessment and rehabilitation of people with disturbed function arising from brain injury, illness or trauma.
> *(Hallet 1993)*

Put simply, neuropsychology is the study of brain–behaviour relationships with its clinical element involving the application of these principles and knowledge to individual patients. In short, while the neurologist assesses the extent of function within the tissues of the central nervous system, it is the neuropsychologist who assesses the individual living within those same tissues.

Some neuropsychologists specialize purely in research, while others specialize in evaluating and treating patients with dysfunctions of the nervous system and have extensive training in the anatomy, physiology, and pathology of the nervous system. In whichever form it takes, neuropsychology is, essentially, the study of brain–behaviour relationships.

Before we embark on a voyage around this most fascinating of specialties, however, we will need to understand a little of the historical background to its development, and make ourselves familiar with the role of the neuropsychologist in the modern healthcare system, the possible reasons for referral to a neuropsychologist, and the scope of assessments and treatments available.

HISTORY OF NEUROPSYCHOLOGY

The use of the term 'neuropsychology' is a relatively recent development. The term was first used in 1949 in the subtitle of a book, *The Organisation of Behaviour: A Neuropsychological Theory* (Hebb 1949). However, the roots of the discipline go back much further to the prehistoric era about 4000 years ago when cranial trephination procedures to treat traumatic head injuries, headaches and seizure disorders were in evidence.

By the time of the early historical era the Egyptians had, for the first time, begun to associate certain brain functions with specific parts of the brain. The earliest written reference to functional lateralization is to be found in the Edwin Smith Surgical Papyrus, dating back to between 2500 and 3000 BC (Breasted 1930). The papyrus, often referred to as the earliest known scientific document, contains anatomical, physiological, pathological, and treatment reports on 48 cases, the first 8 of which deal directly with injuries to the head and brain and include observations on conditions such as lateralized motor dysfunction following trauma in the form of hemiplegia.

Nevertheless, it was not until around 400 BC that the Greek physicians, to whom the works of Hippocrates (circa 425 BC) are now generally attributed, were amongst the first to observe an association between lesions on one side of the brain and motor activity on the contralateral side of the body in studies of epilepsy. Despite these observations, however, Aristotle (384–322 BC) still advanced the so-called cardiocentric viewpoint that it was the heart to which one could localize mental function and that the brain offered only a balancing mechanism for the heart's work.

Galen (AD 130–200), on the other hand, about 400 years later, described in detail the ventricles of the brain and developed a theory of humours flowing through these ventricles and the rest of the body that gave rise to mental functions. This was a theory that was later capitalized upon by Saint Augustine during the 4th Century.

For about 1000 years this theory of mental function persisted with many of the earlier observations of mental function from Aristotle and others being given locations within the ventricles. It was not, however, until the careful anatomy studies of Vesalius (AD 1514–1564) that observation and experiential practice began to win out over the more dogmatic ideas that had persisted since the time of Aristotle. Vesalius was amongst the first to make detailed observations of cerebral anatomy, which although they did not advance our understanding of brain function, did nevertheless advance the cause of empiricism and contribute to our understanding of structural elements.

It was not until the 18th Century, though, that the first global theory of brain function was advanced. The Phrenology theory of Francis Gall (1758–1828) proposed that the development of specific brain areas (known as cerebral organs) resulted in skull prominences that could be analyzed to determine a person's personality and level of intelligence. At the time, Phrenology, which represented the beginnings of the Localizationist doctrine that endures to the present day, was very popular.

Nevertheless, an opposing theory was presented by Pierre Flourens (1794–1867), who asserted that brain functions were not so discreetly localized, and that brain areas worked in concert, producing a general, complex function. This controversy between the Localizationists and Holists was not to be resolved until studies were undertaken in the 19th Century by neurologists such as Broca.

Paul Broca, a French surgeon and anthropologist was, in 1861, introduced to a Monsieur Leborgne (nicknamed 'Tan' after the patient's only verbal utterance). Leborgne was admitted to Broca's surgery service for treatment of cellulitis. However, he was also an epileptic who had lost the ability to speak at around the age of 30 years and in his 40s had developed a right-sided paresis.

Unfortunately, Leborgne died shortly after meeting with Broca. At autopsy, however, it was discovered that this patient had lesions of the left frontal lobe. Broca presented this case to the next meeting of the Society of Anthropology in Paris as evidence supporting the Localizationist doctrine and observed that there was some sort of relationship between speech and the left frontal area (Broca 1861).

Soon thereafter there began a more systematic study of what Broca termed 'aphemia', a term later to be replaced by the expression 'aphasia' by which we know the condition today.

By 1874, Carl Wernike, a German neurologist, had published a paper that suggested there was a clinical separation between the motor and sensory aspects of speech, or what are termed today expressive and receptive aphasia, in what was now increasingly referred to as the 'dominant' hemisphere of the brain after the earlier introduction of the concept by the English neurologist, John Hughlings Jackson.

Jackson proposed that the two apparently symmetrical hemispheres of the brain played differing roles in function. Jackson proposed that the left cerebral hemisphere was responsible for mediating verbal activity and the right for visuoperceptive, visuospatial, and visuoconstructive functions, although, at the time, many of Jackson's observations concerning the right cerebral hemisphere were largely overlooked. Nevertheless, the modern doctrine of component process localization was born and with it the concept that complex mental functions might, in fact, represent the combined processing of a number of subcomponent processes represented in widely different areas of the brain.

Towards the end of the 19th Century the discoveries concerning brain function were coming thick and fast, when in 1887, Korsakoff noted a relationship between memory function and toxic metabolic states, with a number of these early cases involving patients who were chronic alcohol abusers. Similar observations were being made by Wernicke at around the same time and it soon became clear that the cases seen by Korsakoff and Wernicke were essentially different examples of the same disorder. Thus, it was discovered that a nutritional deficiency could result in damage to the structures of the brain involved with the recall of new information. This cluster of symptoms we now refer to as Wernicke–Korsakoff syndrome.

At the beginning of the 20th Century, Hugo Leipmann further reinforced the Localizationist perspective with his observations of apraxia, a disorder of purposeful movement, demonstrating that while such disorders were not due to an inability to comprehend speech they were, nevertheless, associated with damage to the left cerebral hemisphere.

It was at the beginning of the 20th Century that the concept of a cerebral dominance for the functions of the left hemisphere over the subordinate and largely silent right hemisphere began to influence research. However, no sooner had the concept of cerebral dominance become established than evidence began to emerge that suggested that the right cerebral hemisphere was, in fact, possessed of a number of specialized abilities of its own.

Initially, these challenges to the dominance of the left hemisphere were observed in research into deficits arising from simultaneous injuries to both sides of the brain. For example, early work on the pathophysiology of spatial disorientation and topographic memory disturbance suggested that such deficits were not an exclusive feature of left hemisphere damage but related to a bilateral involvement (Holmes & Horrax 1919). Similarly, it was noted by Wolpert (1924) that simultangosia, an inability to perceive more than one stimulus or more than one aspect of a stimulus at a time, was another syndrome which appeared to manifest itself when damage occurred to both the left and right hemispheres.

Later, however, it became apparent that well-defined, unilateral lesions of the right cerebral hemisphere could produce their own profound changes in observable behaviour. For example, one of the first large-scale psychometric assessments of patients with brain damage conducted during the 1930s (Weisenberg & McBride 1935) revealed, as might be expected, that lesions of the left cerebral hemisphere resulted in poor performance on tests of verbal ability. However, it was also noted that patients with damage to the right hemisphere were consistently poorer on tests of non-verbal ability, suggesting that the right hemisphere played a specialized role in visuospatial functions.

Further developing on these and other early studies, more intensive research during the 1950s and 1960s began to radically alter the accepted profile of functioning within the brain. For example, it was proposed that the right cerebral hemisphere played a significant role in melodic processing (Kimura 1964), while it was also suggested that the right hemisphere was more specialized for visual memory and face recognition (Milner 1968).

As time has progressed and our understanding of brain function has been enhanced by newer and more detailed research we have come to learn that neither hemisphere is absolutely dominant and that each is, in fact, specialized for different functions. For instance, language, the first of the areas of brain function to be investigated in detail, now appears to be represented in both the left and right hemispheres, with Eisenson (1962) and Critchley (1962) first postulating the concept of a right hemisphere contribution to language processing, and with later work appearing to confirm this contribution in terms of expression, reception, and comprehension (Mackenzie et al 1997).

Historically, then, both the Localizationist and the Holistic camps have enjoyed popular acceptance, with the former predominant for the better part of the 20th Century. However, as our understanding of the nature of cerebral functioning has increased, so we have observed a synthesis of the two positions, with neither hemisphere holding an entirely dominant position, but rather both contributing to different specialized functions in the form of a systemic whole. It was these steps forward, then, and many others that shifted our fundamental understanding of the brain and that led ultimately to a need to understand and accurately measure its functions, which finally paved the way for the emergence of neuropsychology in the 1940s, 1950s and 1960s as a distinct and identifiable discipline within the neurosciences.

Nevertheless, this embryonic specialty, despite a sound foundation, was not fully established until quite recently. To get a flavour of just how new neuropsychology is, we need only look at its development within the psychological community as a whole. To illustrate, the International Neuropsychology Society (INS) was only founded in 1967, whilst the American Psychological Association (APA) only granted separate divisional specialty status to Clinical Neuropsychology during 1996, a divisional specialty not granted to members of the British Psychological Society (BPS) until 1999.

THE MODERN ROLE OF THE NEUROPSYCHOLOGIST

Building on this valuable history of research and discovery, then, what of the role of the modern neuropsychologist? Despite its relative youth, neuropsychology today has firmly established itself between the fields of medicine and psychology. It provides assessment and treatments for patients suffering with a wide variety of conditions such as stroke, head injury, dementia and depressive pseudodementia, multiple sclerosis, Parkinson's disease, Huntington's disease, epilepsy and pseudoseizures, developmental disorder, and the variety of conditions arising from metabolic disorder or exposure to toxic substances.

Given the recent advances in neuro-imaging technology you would be forgiven for wondering what purpose the neuropsychologist fulfills in an era of single photon emission computed tomography (SPECT) and positron emission tomography (PET). However, there are many factors that cannot be evaluated through classical means (try examining personality, emotion or short-term memory on the next magnetic resonance image (MRI), computed tomography (CT) scan or eletroencephalogram (EEG) you come across and you will begin to understand why). Therefore, the task of the neuropsychologist has become, in some senses, more complicated as advances in technology have led to an increased expectation in the sensitivity and specificity of the neuropsychological measures used.

The first task of the neuropsychologist, therefore, is to make an accurate assessment of the patient and their various deficits. In order to provide an accurate report of the presence of a given disorder, the degree to which this disorder may affect psychological functioning, and its likely course, the neuropsychologist must employ a wide range of assessment measures (Green 1997).

Initially, these assessment tools were not designed specifically to measure damage to the brain. For example, amongst the earliest tests to be utilized by neuropsychologists was the Wechsler Adult Intelligence Scale or WAIS. However, while this test was originally designed to assess intellectual capacity in academic or vocational settings, it soon became apparent that it, and its various successors, also had uses in the evaluation of impaired cognition such as that which can accompany insults to the central nervous system. Later, more specific tests were developed and, as we will see later, either grouped together in fixed batteries or kept as stand alone single instruments, with some neuropsychologists preferring the use of the fixed battery and others choosing to use individual tests as the presentation of the patient dictated.

From whichever stand-point, however, the neuropsychological assessment broadly falls into four main areas:

1. *Diagnosis*: determination of the nature of a problem. For example, if someone complains of a short-term memory deficit, it is important to be able to discriminate between organic impairment and, for example, the psychological disturbance of cognition often seen in depression.
2. *Delineation*: to determine the nature and degree of any neuropsychological impairment.
3. *Measurement of change*: to determine the degree of change in function over time. This may represent measurement of improvement with a given treatment or, alternatively, the measurement of rate of decline in a progressively degenerating disorder.
4. *Treatment planning*: the accurate assessment of neuropsychological disturbance, providing a platform for treatment.

Based on the results of the assessment, the neuropsychologist will then endeavour to provide support and advice to both patients and carers, and begin to develop, where appropriate, a programme of rehabilitative cognitive retraining. Overall, these interventions are aimed at reducing distress, increasing understanding and control and, as a consequence, providing a means by which patients can appropriately express their emotional reactions. Once again, these treatments can be subdivided into three broad areas:

1. *Information*: the provision of information often helps both patients and carers to develop an understanding, and to some degree an accommodation, of the cognitive and emotional difficulties associated with the patient's condition.
2. *Support*: the development of any severe illness can have a sudden, unexpected, and tremendously pervasive effect on an individual's life, creating psychological and emotional imbalance. However, in the case of neuropsychological disorders, the effect is perhaps amplified because it strikes at the very core of what defines our lives – our memories, personalities and so on. Informed psychotherapeutic intervention to provide emotional support and assistance in the adaptation/adjustment process, therefore, is of the utmost importance.
3. *Cognitive rehabilitation*: the amelioration of disturbed cognitive functions and the restoration of impaired skills through the stimulation of those systems which demonstrate impairment, the development of intact skills, and training in the means through which a specific impairment can be compensated for or minimized.

Referral to a neuropsychologist may be initiated for a number of specific reasons. Again, however, these can generally be divided into four broad categories:

1. *Diagnosis*: neuropsychological assessment can be useful in discriminating between psychiatric and neurological symptoms, identifying a

possible neurological disorder, helping to distinguish between different neurological conditions, and providing behavioural data for localizing the site of damage. For example, a neuropsychologist might be referred a patient with symptoms of cognitive disturbance in order to determine the presence of a cerebral dysfunction in the absence of clear structural anatomical evidence.

2. *Patient care and planning*: providing information on a patient's strengths and weakness, areas of vulnerability and likely performance in different circumstances, provides a valuable profile from which more effective treatment planning can be derived. For instance, a patient who has suffered a cerebrovascular event (CVE) or closed head injury (CHI) might suffer difficulties with memory such that this makes it difficult to comply with a medication regimen or return to the workplace. A neuropsychological assessment under these circumstances can provide useful information on the type and extent of the memory disorder, the likelihood and degree of recovery that might be anticipated, and the possible vulnerabilities of the patient in different situations.
3. *Rehabilitation and treatment evaluation*: neuropsychological assessment can provide a powerful evaluation of the efficacy of ongoing treatments or rehabilitative interventions, can help to further optimize treatment efficacy, and can examine questions such as treatment compliance.
4. *Medicolegal evaluation*: increasingly, neuropsychologists are called upon to contribute to legal proceedings. This might involve the documentation of the presence, nature, and extent of cerebral dysfunction in personal injury cases; the determination of the capacity of patients to defend themselves in legal cases; or the evaluation of organic factors in mitigation.

SUMMARY

As we have seen, then, the goal of neuropsychology is to understand the relationship between brain and behaviour. The discipline has a long and varied history dating back to the time of the Egyptians and Greeks, through Broca's landmark work in the area of language, Gall's interpretation of cerebral activity giving rise to skull prominences, Hughlings Jackson's observations on the lateralization of function, and ultimately the synthesis of the Localizationist and Holistic approaches of the 18th Century into our modern understanding of the brain and its functions.

The modern neuropsychologist, then, in the role of the scientist–practitioner, continues to expand on this historical knowledge base, researching that which is still unclear whilst assessing and treating those unfortunate enough to have suffered damage to the brain. In so doing, the neuropsychologist provides insights into diagnosis, the nature and extent of impairment, the qualitative impact of damage, and the ways and means in which patient care might be enhanced; provides information and informed support to patients and carers, and offers specific treatments aimed at the improvement of impaired cognition.

REFERENCES

Breasted J H 1930 The Edwin Smith Surgical Papyrus. University of Chicago Press, Chicago

Broca P 1861 Nouvelle observation d'aphemie produite par une lesion de la posterieure des deuxieme et troisieme circonvolutions frontale. Bulletin de la Societé Anotomique de Paris 6:398–407

Critchley M 1962 Speech and speech loss in relation to duality in the brain. In: Mountcastle V B (ed) Interhemispheric relations and cerebral dominance. Johns Hopkins University Press, Baltimore

Eisenson J 1962, Language and intellectual modifications associated with right cerebral damage. Journal of Speech and Language 5:49–53

Green C 1997 Psychometric tests. In: Goodwill C, Chamberlain M, Evans C (eds) Rehabilitation of the physically disabled adult, 2nd edn. Stanley Thornes, Cheltenham

Hallett S 1993 Neuropsychology. In: Morgan G, Butler S (eds) Seminars in basic neurosciences. Gaskell, London

Hebb D O 1949 The organisation of behaviour: a neuropsychological theory. Wiley, New York

Holmes G, Horrax G 1919 Disturbances of spatial orientation and visual attention, with loss of stereoscopic vision. Archives of Neurology and Psychiatry 1:385–407

Kimura D 1964 Left-right differences in the perception of melodies. Quarterly Journal of Experimental Psychology 16:355–358

Mackenzie C, Begg T, Brady M et al 1997 The effects on verbal communication skills of right hemisphere stroke in middle age. Aphasiology 11:929–945

Milner B 1968 Visual recognition and recall after temporal lobe excision in man. Neuropsychologia 6:191–209

Weisenberg T, McBride K E 1935 Aphasia: a clinical and psychological study. Commonwealth Fund, New York

Wolpert I 1924 Die simultagnosie: Störung der gesamtauffassung, Zeitschrift für die gesamte. Neurologie und Psychiatrie 93:397–415

FURTHER READING

Haligan P W, Kischka U, Marshall J C 2003 Handbook of clinical neuropsychology. Oxford University Press, Oxford

Martin G N 1998 Human neuropsychology. Prentice Hall Europe, London

Neuroanatomy

2

OVERVIEW

As with all complex mechanisms, the central nervous system (CNS) comprises a number of subdivisions. Some of these are easily visualized; for example the division between the brain and spinal cord. Some of them are superimposed upon the tissues by neuroscientists to provide a topographical reference point; for instance the division between the temporal and frontal lobe. Yet others divide the brain into areas grouped by similarities in their cellular structure.

In practice, neuropsychological diagnosis involves the collection of data from histories, behavioural observations and test performance to provide insights into the type and degree of functional disability and, inevitably, this will often involve some degree of localization. In simple terms, for example, we know that in the majority of right-handed people, the motor aspects of speech are represented in an area of the left frontal lobe known as Broca's area. Thus, if there is a problem in motor speech behaviour we can deduce the involvement of this area and can often observe an associated weakness or paralysis of the right arm.

In reality, however, the brain is a sophisticated and intricate system, the functional aspects of which are not so easily localized to a single area. To illustrate, some patients with the same obvious signs of left hemisphere motor involvement in the form of a weakness or paralysis of the right arm are able to verbalize without difficulty, while others have demonstrated well-defined brain lesions on computed tomography (CT) scanning but with no apparent symptoms. Indeed, at its most extreme, a small percentage of left-handed people may have a complete reversal of this pattern of functional localization, with expressive speech represented on the right and not the left side of the brain.

Clearly, therefore, the localization of function to specific brain areas has both its uses and limitations. It can prove an invaluable means of data transmission in cases of common patterns of neurobehavioural disability associated with well-understood conditions that tend to involve similar anatomical structures, as long as we are cautious and remember that numerous exceptions to the accepted rules exist.

With this codicil in mind, then, we will take a journey into the major divisions of the brain and examine each of the main structures in some detail.

We will acquaint ourselves with some of the terminology used to describe these structures and then, in the next chapter, turn our attention to some of the more common functional results of damage.

TERMINOLOGY

Sadly, the considerable terminology associated with neuroanatomy can, at first glance, appear bewildering and confusing. Often it serves to discourage those new to the neurosciences and can act as an effective soporific to those embroiled in its study. However, as we shall see later, just a handful of these specific terms can prove useful in furthering our understanding.

Before we commence examination of the various areas of the brain, we will take a brief look at some of the more common terms used. For simplicity the more frequently used terms appear in Box 2.1.

The direction of structures within the brain is described according to their axis; that is to say, where the structures fall in relation to lines drawn through the spinal cord and brain. Thus, a structure that lies at the back of the head, for example the occipital lobe, may be described as posterior to an imagined

Box 2.1 Common anatomical and functional terminology

A-	Complete loss, e.g. aphasia
Afferent	Structures such as neurons conveying information to a given area
Anterior	At the front
Bilateral	On both sides
Caudal	Towards the spinal cord
Contralateral	On the opposite side
Coronal	Vertical section through the brain dividing the front from the back
Distal	Near
Dorsal	The top or back of
Dys-	Partial loss, e.g. dyspraxia
Efferent	Structures such as neurons conveying information away from a given area
Gyrus	A raised area on the surface of the brain (plural gyri)
Inferior	Below
Ipsilateral	On the same side
Lateral	Towards the side
Lobe	An area of the brain usually associated with prominent sulci
Medial	Towards the mid-line
Mid-line	The line dividing the right and left cerebral hemispheres
Posterior	At the back
Proximal	Far
Rostral	Away from the spinal cord
Sagittal	Vertical section through the brain dividing left and right cerebral hemispheres
Sulcus	Fissure between two gyri (plural sulci)
Superior	Above
Unilateral	On one side
Ventral	Towards the top or front
Ventricle	Space in the brain through which cerebrospinal fluid circulates (CSF)

line drawn through the middle of the brain, while a structure that lies towards the front of the head, for example the frontal lobe, is said to be anterior to this same imaginary line.

Other structures can be positionally described in a similar manner. For example, the temporal lobe is more anterior than the occipital lobe but inferior to the parietal lobe; or, more informally, it is more forward than the occipital lobe and below the parietal lobe.

Initially, such language can be quite confusing, especially when terms are joined together to form polysyllabic expressions. However, with a little perseverance they can be mastered and offer an advantage, although not an essential one, in terms of a fuller understanding of neuroanatomy.

MAJOR DIVISIONS OF THE NERVOUS SYSTEM

In this introduction to basic neuroanatomy, we will look briefly at the building blocks of the nervous system, the neurons, and their place in the peripheral nervous system (PNS) and the CNS. We will then focus on the CNS and the major structures of the brain. This concentration on the CNS does not, of course, imply that other structures within the nervous system are not as important as those of the brain itself. However, to put this organization of the text into perspective, it will be remembered that the more common observations made in neuropsychology will involve the CNS.

To this end, then, we will first look at the structure of the neuron and the various divisions of the PNS. Next we will explore the spinal cord, brainstem and cerebellum, the subcortical territories, examine the major anatomical subdivisions of the cortex, look at the brain's blood supply, the ventricular system, and finally examine the various outer protective coverings of the brain.

Neuron

The nervous system as a whole is composed of millions of nerve cells called neurons (from the Greek, meaning nerve). The neurons are highly specialized cells, transmitting electrochemical impulses to and from all parts of the body. All neurons have a cell body which performs all the basic metabolic processes (such as the synthesis of proteins), and which surrounds a central nucleus containing the cell's DNA.

In addition, the neurons possess two types of structural extension known as axons and dendrites. Axons are long, slender fibres that carry impulses from the cell body. The axons can range in length from fractions of an inch in the brain to 2 or more feet long in the spinal cord and PNS. To insulate them, axons are sheathed in a layer of myelin (Fig. 2.1).

Normally, this myelin layer does not form a continuous sheath along the entire length of an axon but is broken in regular intervals by junctions called the nodes of Ranvier. Axons divide at their ends into telondendria to form bulb-like structures known as terminal buttons. These terminal buttons, in turn, release chemical substances called neurotransmitters that enable nerve impulses to travel from one neuron to the next.

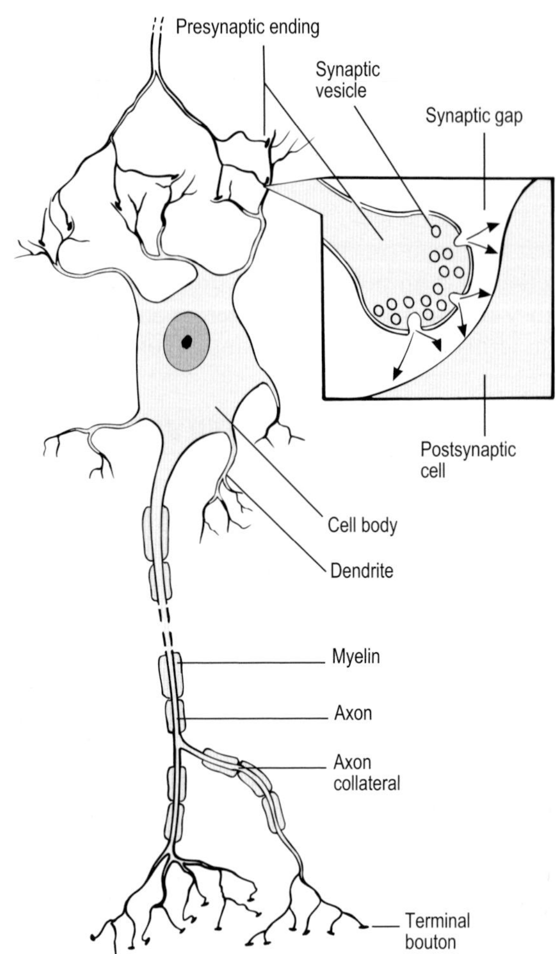

Fig. 2.1 The neuron. (From Crossman & Neary 2000, p 2)

The dendrites (from the Greek, meaning tree), on the other hand, are thin, branched extensions of the neuron receiving impulses from adjacent cells and conveying these to the cell body. Dendrites receive impulses from other neurons via neurotransmitters across the synapse, a receiving and transmission area containing both the axon's terminal buttons and the dendrite, and a synaptic cleft, a small space between the receiving dendrites and the transmitting axons (typically a gap of about 5 millionths of an inch).

There are three main types of neuron within the nervous system: afferent neurons, carrying impulses to the CNS from receptor sites around the body; efferent neurons, carrying impulses from the CNS to the body; and interneurons, which reside only in the CNS and provide an intermediate role between afferent and efferent neurons.

Peripheral nervous system

The peripheral nervous system (PNS) conducts impulses to and from the CNS; that is, the brain and spinal cord. Neurons in the PNS have their cell bodies within the CNS, but the greater part of their length lies outside it. The PNS consists of neurons with both myelinated and unmyelinated axons (Fig. 2.2).

Containing both efferent or motor neurons and afferent or sensory neurons, the PNS is divided into two parts: the somatic nervous system (SNS) and the autonomic nervous system (ANS). The SNS consists of 12 pairs of cranial nerves and 31 pairs of spinal nerves, receiving sensory impulses and sending motor impulses. The ANS, meanwhile, innervates the body's organs and glands, conveying impulses to and from the CNS, meeting the needs of those automatic functions that we are rarely aware of, such as heart activity and the release of hormones. The ANS is further subdivided into the sympathetic nervous system and the parasympathetic nervous system, which are responsible for the stimulation or the retardation of this system.

Spinal cord

The spinal cord occupies the upper two-thirds of the canal formed by the vertebrae. The vertebral column itself consists of 24 individual vertebrae as well as fused vertebrae in the sacral and coccygeal regions. In the centre of each vertebra are spaces through which the spinal cord passes. At its upper extremity, it is continuous with the brain stem and neurons exiting the bones surrounding the CNS; the spinal and cranial nerves are considered part of the PNS.

Like the brain, the spinal cord is made up of grey matter and white matter. The grey matter is located centrally and contains the cell bodies of neurons. The white matter surrounds the grey matter and contains both the ascending and descending, and sensory and motor pathways.

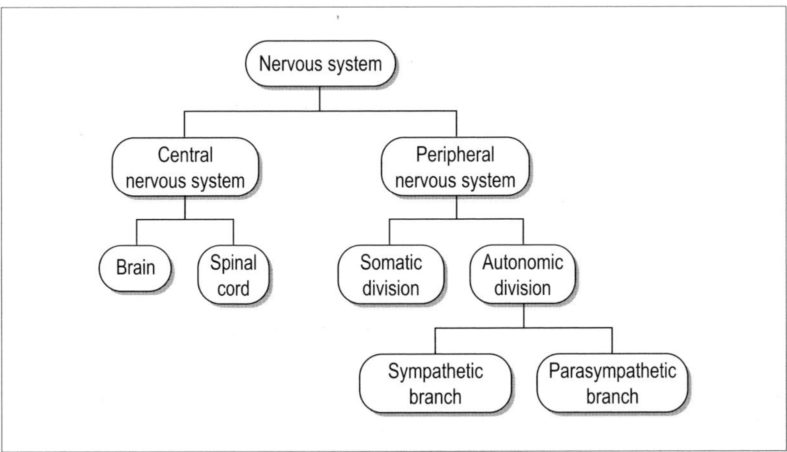

Fig. 2.2 The organization of the nervous system.

Brainstem and subcortical system

There are six main structures at the core of the brain and we will look at each of these in relation to its anatomical positioning.

The brainstem forms a continuation of the spinal cord and comprises the medulla, reticular formation, pons and cerebellum (Fig. 2.3).

The medulla is directly superior to the spinal cord and, indeed, many of its functions are similar to that of the spinal cord. However, it also contains a number of nuclei or nerve centres giving rise to most but not all of the cranial nerves. It is also at the level of the medulla that motor fibres from one side of the body cross over onto the opposite side, giving rise to the contralateral control of the left side of the body with the right side of the brain and vice versa. Finally, the medulla controls a great many vital life support functions such as respiration, blood pressure, body temperature and heart rate and, therefore, it is for this reason that damage at this level can often prove fatal.

The pons (a Latin term for bridge) and cerebellum are structures that lie high on the brainstem and together they regulate both postural and kinaesthetic movement. The pons lies superior to the medulla and anterior to the cerebellum. It acts as an important centre for certain types of eye movement and balance control and acts as a convergence, relay, and comparison centre for the auditory information received at the ear.

The cerebellum (a Latin term for little brain), meanwhile, lies posterior to the medulla and pons and is important for the regulation of muscle tone and the direction of motor activity. As a part of the motor system, the cerebellum is involved in the creation of even body movements and the control of small deviations in the paths of movement. It is also involved in the learning of skilled movements such as the playing of musical instruments. Thus, while damage in this area will not cause paralysis it will tend to produce an interference with the production of precise motor control, causing jerky or spastic movement and speech difficulties, as well as a disruption of equilibrium.

Above the pons lies the midbrain within which reside the inferior and superior colliculus, which play a role in our orientation to both visual and auditory stimuli. The superior colliculus allows us to perceive and orient to large moving objects in our peripheral vision and also helps to guide the eyes to place objects in the central visual field. The inferior colliculus, like the pons, acts as a relay point for auditory information and, along with the action of other structures, helps us to orient our heads and eyes to significant auditory stimuli.

Finally, in the core of the brainstem lies a cluster of nerve cells and fibres collectively known as the reticular formation. The different groupings of these neurons play a variety of roles in the maintenance of muscle tone, the mediation of postural reflexes and muscle activity, and prepare the cortex for the arrival of sensory input. Parts of this formation, known as the reticular activating system, or RAS, are involved in the regulation of wakefulness, whereby consciousness and alertness are maintained through the action of pathways which detect incoming sensory information and pass activating signals to the cortex. Thus damage in this area can lead to sleep disorders

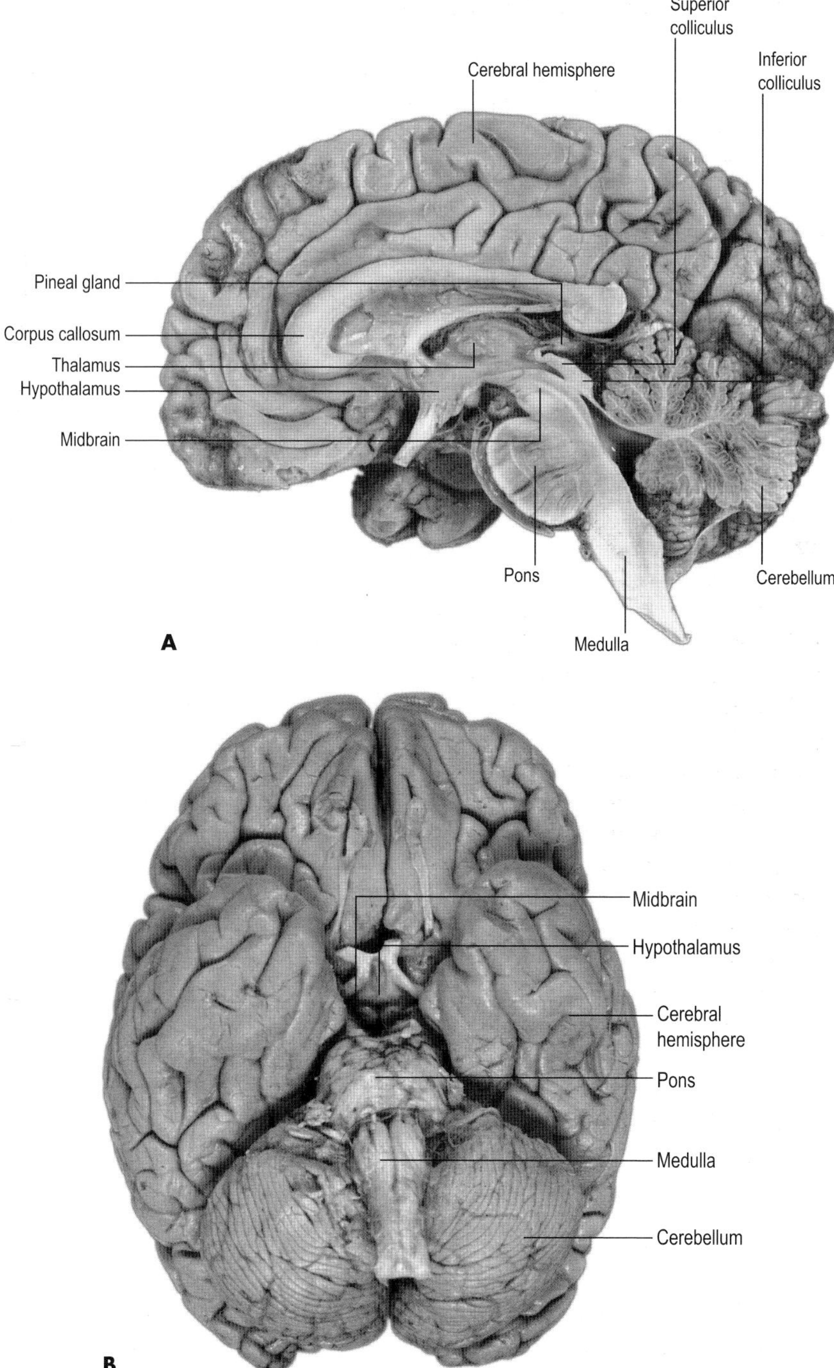

Fig. 2.3 The brainstem and cerebellum. (From Crossman & Neary 2000, p 9)

and disturbances of consciousness and responsiveness leading to drowsiness, somnolence, hypersomnolence or coma.

Above the brainstem and underlying the cortex are the main subcortical systems: the limbic system, basal ganglia, thalamus, and hypothalamus. Situated atop the brainstem, the thalamus acts as a relay point for sensory information entering the cortex and motor information leaving it. The thalamus has numerous elaborate connections with the cortex and almost all other parts of the CNS. Thus damage in this area can result in serious neurological impairment.

Below the thalamus at the base of the brain lies the hypothalamus. It is closely connected with the limbic system and has a close relationship with the hormonal or endocrine system. The role of the hypothalamus is in homeostasis or the control of behaviours which help to maintain bodily equilibrium or need satisfaction. For example, the hypothalamus is involved in feeding and drinking behaviour, respiratory function, body temperature, sexual behaviour and emotional responses.

The limbic system and its associated structures were once believed to be an integration point for emotional information within the nervous system but they are now known to play a much more complex role in a variety of functions. These structures include the amygdala, anterior hypothalamus, cingulated cortex, anterior thalamus, the mamilliary bodies, the septal nuclei and the hippocampus (Fig. 2.4).

This complex system consists of a network of intricate pathways connecting a number of cortical and subcortical systems important in memory, emotion, learning, cortical arousal, motor control, reproductive behaviour and sleep. The septal nuclei, for instance, have been implicated in the experience of pleasure (Olds & Milner 1954), while the amygdala is thought to play

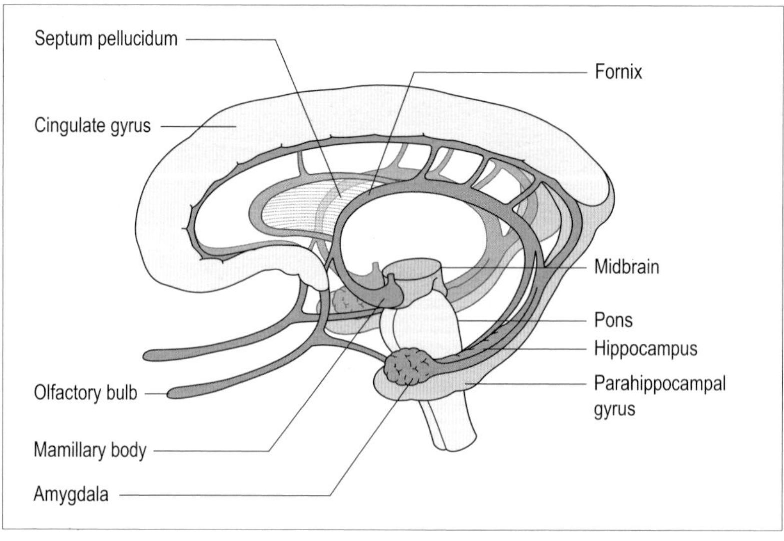

Fig. 2.4 The subcortical structures. (After Smart 2001)

a role in aggressive responses (Chozick 1986) and anxiety and fear (Aggleton 1992).

The basal ganglia, overlying the thalamus, again consist of another subset of subcortical structures comprising: the caudate nucleus, putamen, globus pallidus, and substantia nigra. These structures are important in motor control, with damage or degeneration in this area leading to difficulties characterized by involuntary movements, changes in posture, and increases or decreases in muscle tone. For example, with damage to the globus pallidus, an involuntary twisting and turning of the limbs is observed, while damage to the caudate nucleus and putamen leads to resting tremors such those seen in Parkinson's disease.

Cerebral cortex

The cortex or neocortex, so called because of its relatively recent evolutionary development, is the most immediately obvious structure when we think of brain tissue. It has an average surface area of 2.5 square feet and consists of convolutions called sulci and gyri which allow for this surface area and thereby allow for its development within the confined space of the skull. Indeed, if more substantial brain development were to take place in utero, the skull and the underlying brain would be too large to pass through the birth canal.

Each individual brain, whilst possessing many common features such as the placement of the lobes, also possesses a certain uniqueness of gyral pattern making no two cerebral cortices exactly the same. When a sulcus is particularly deep it is known as a fissure and it is these that serve as landmarks in defining the borders of major functional areas. Figure 2.5 shows these major divisions. The first and most obvious is the midline longitudinal fissure dividing the brain into two hemispheres, connected through a thick band of fibres known as the corpus callosum. Next is the central fissure, sometimes referred to as the Rolandic fissure, separating each hemisphere into anterior and posterior sections. Generally speaking, areas in front of this division play a role in motor processing, while those behind tend to play more of a role in sensory processing. Finally, each individual hemisphere is further subdivided by the lateral or Sylvian fissure separating the dorsal from the ventral.

Together, these fissures not only provide landmarks for anatomical examination but also act as divisions in each hemisphere between the four individual lobes. Thus the area anterior to or in front of the central fissure is known as the frontal lobe. The area inferior to or below the Sylvian fissure is known as the temporal lobe. The area posterior to or behind the central fissure and superior to or above the Sylvian fissure is known as the parietal lobe. Finally, the area posterior to or behind all of these is known as the occipital lobe.

Blood supply and the blood–brain barrier

Although the brain only accounts for some 2% of the mass of the whole body, it requires around 20% of the blood supply. Blood is supplied to the brain via

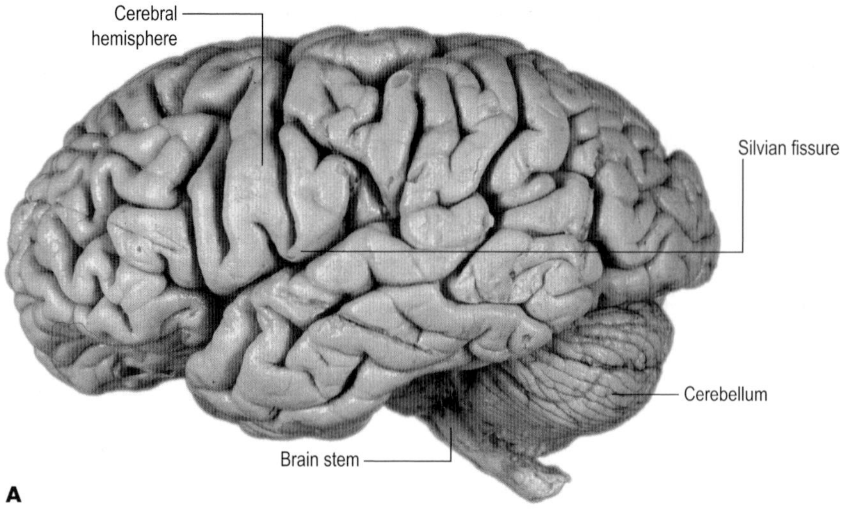

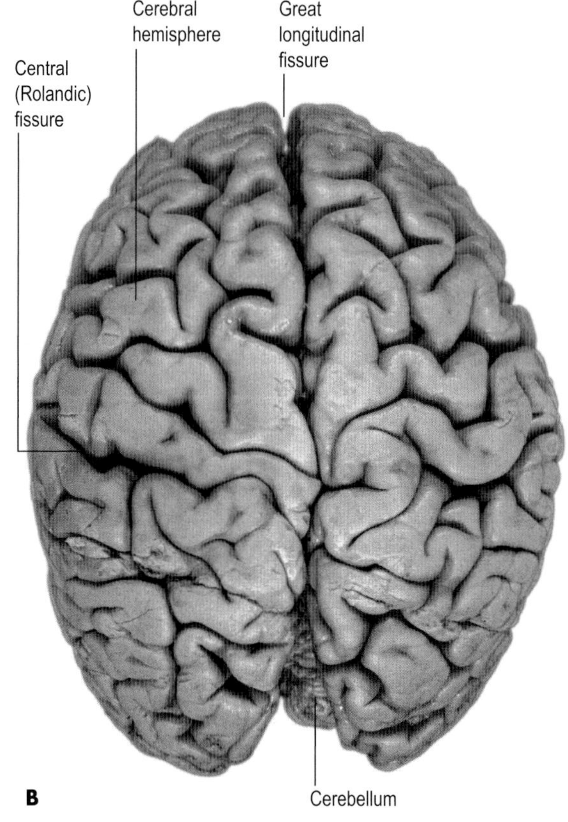

Fig. 2.5 The brain and major anatomical divisions. (Adapted from Crossman & Neary 2000, p 9)

the internal carotid artery, providing a flow of oxygenated blood to the cortex, and the vertebral artery, providing a flow to the brainstem and cerebellum.

The carotid artery enters the skull and divides into the ophthalmic, anterior cerebral and middle cerebral arteries, with smaller divisions from these vessels supplying most of the cortex. The vertebral artery forms the basilar artery at the level of the pons which, in turn, branches to the medulla, pons, and cerebellum. The basilar artery divides at the top of the pons to form the posterior cerebral arteries, supplying blood to the occipital cortex and inferior temporal lobe.

Joining the middle cerebral artery and the posterior cerebral artery is the posterior communicating artery; while a similar vessel called the anterior communicating artery joins the anterior cerebral arteries. Forming a link between these anterior and posterior supply systems, this group of communicating vessels, collectively known as the Circle of Willis, allows collateral circulation to take place when another vessel becomes occluded (Fig. 2.6). Veins in the brain are classified as external, internal or cerebellar. These empty into a system of deep folds in the dura mater called venous sinuses. For stable function to take place within the brain, not only does the blood supply have to remain constant, since even a small interruption can have serious consequences for both cortical and subcortical structures, but there must also be a controlled flow of molecules to the brain from the blood.

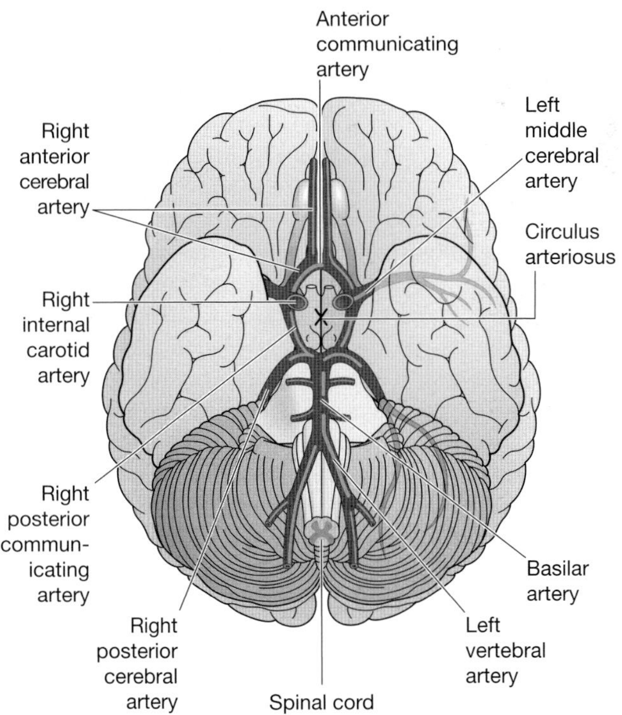

Fig. 2.6 The brain's blood supply. (From Waugh & Grant 2001, p 100)

Protecting the brain from all but the most necessary substances such as glucose, oxygen and water, and preventing toxins or pathogens from entering, is the blood–brain barrier. Lining the walls of the capillaries supplying the brain tissues is a layer of tightly packed endothelial cells that impede the flow of toxins or pathogens from the blood to the brain. Similarly, the blood–brain barrier serves to protect the tissues from invasion by the very blood that transports its nutrients to it, since blood itself is autotoxaemic (self-poisoning) to the delicate tissues of the brain.

Such a structure has obvious beneficial qualities protecting the brain from toxins, but this itself poses a further problem since the molecular structure of the immune system's antibodies, lymphocytes and phagocytes means they also have difficulty in crossing this barrier. The immune system, then, is largely prevented from protecting the CNS against infection and the brain relies heavily, therefore, on the blood–brain barrier's ability to block the entry of infectious agents.

Unfortunately, however, while this arrangement often works well, when infection does occur as in meningitis (a swelling of the brain's protective membranes), the blood–brain barrier makes the direct treatment of such illness difficult since the molecular structure of, for example, antibiotics such as penicillin makes it ineffective. Thus, while many molecules will cross this barrier, for example oxygen, glucose, carbon dioxide, nicotine, and morphine, many substances will not.

Ventricular system and cerebrospinal fluid

The lateral ventricles are cavities in each of the cerebral hemispheres. These cavities contain cerebral spinal fluid and each is divided into five portions: the anterior horn, ventricular body, collateral trigone, the inferior horn, and the posterior horn. The third ventricle is narrow and located midline, while the fourth ventricle lies above the pons and medulla (Fig. 2.7).

The entire surface of the CNS, that is the brain and spinal cord, is bathed in cerebrospinal fluid. CSF, a colourless liquid composed mainly of sodium chloride, with smaller amounts of protein, potassium and glucose, is produced by a structure called the choroid plexus located in the lateral, third, and fourth ventricles. Its total volume is around 125 mL (Fig. 2.8).

CSF flows from the lateral ventricles to the third ventricle through the interventricular foramen, also known as the foramen of Monro. The third and fourth ventricles are connected to each other by the cerebral aqueduct, also known as the Aqueduct of Sylvius. It then flows into the subarachnoid space through the foramina of Luschka and Magendie.

Absorption of the CSF into the blood stream takes place in the superior sagittal sinus through structures called the arachnoid villi. When CSF pressure is greater than the venous pressure, it will flow into the blood stream. However, when CSF pressure is less than venous pressure, the arachnoid villi act to prevent blood from passing into the ventricular system.

The CSF has four main functions. It:

- protects the brain from damage by acting as a buffer to mechanical trauma

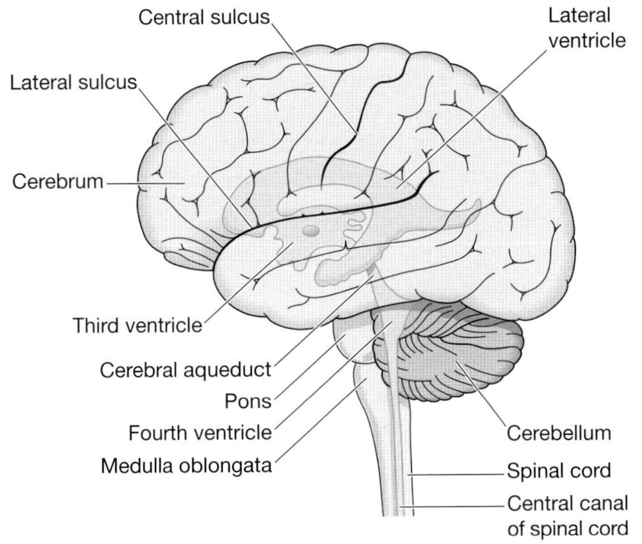

Fig. 2.7 The ventricular system. (From Waugh & Grant 2001, p 148)

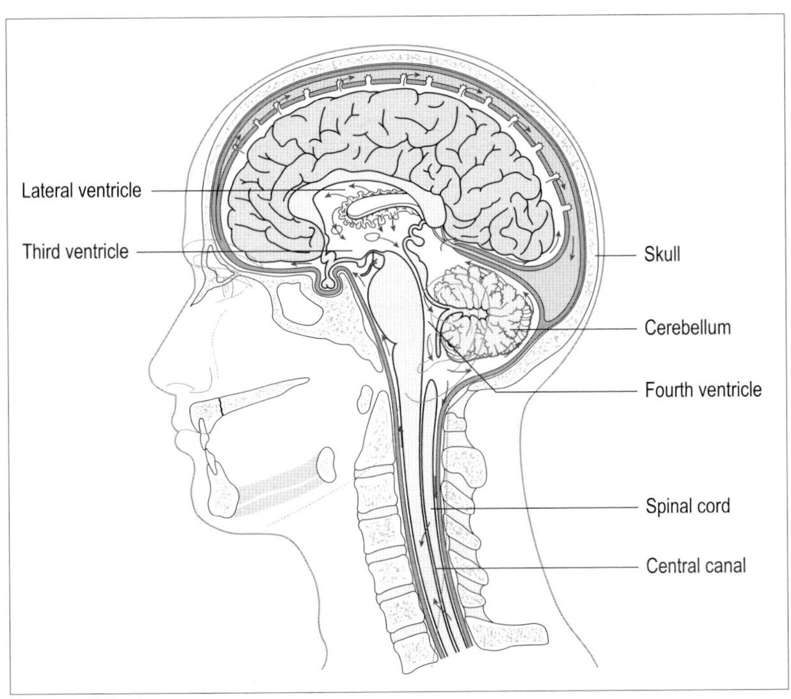

Fig. 2.8 The cerebrospinal fluid. (After Smart 2001)

- acts as a support medium for the brain, reducing pressure at the base of the brain
- provides a unidirectional flow for waste products and other substances away from the brain
- provides a medium for the transport of hormones to other areas of the brain.

In some conditions, CSF produced at a rate of approximately 400 to 500 mL per day can build up in the ventricles. An over-production or an obstruction to flow can, therefore, lead to the condition of hydrocephalus and enlargement of the ventricles.

Protective coverings of the brain

The first and most obvious of these protective layers is the skull (Fig. 2.9). Composed of the maxilla, frontal, ethmoid, sphenoid, temporal, parietal and occipital bones, the skull encloses the brain and, except for the lower jawbone or mandible, does not articulate. It contains various foramina that permit the passage of major arteries, veins and cranial nerves. The largest of these, known as the foramen magnum, allows for the continuation of the brainstem down into the spinal cord.

In newborn infants, the skull is approximately 25% of adult size and reaches approximately 75% of adult size by the end of the 1st year of life. At this stage the skull is composed of relatively thin and pliable bones separated by fibrous tissues known as sutures and these, where most bone growth occurs, do not completely knit until approximately 8 years of age.

Inside the skull and directly overlying the brain are three layers of tissue collectively called the meninges (Fig. 2.10). The outer layer of the meninges,

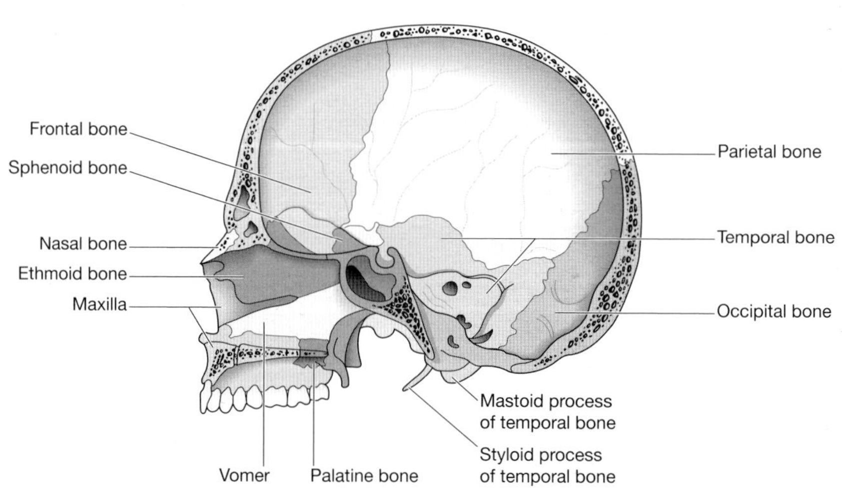

Fig. 2.9 The bones of the skull. (From Waugh & Grant 2001, p 49)

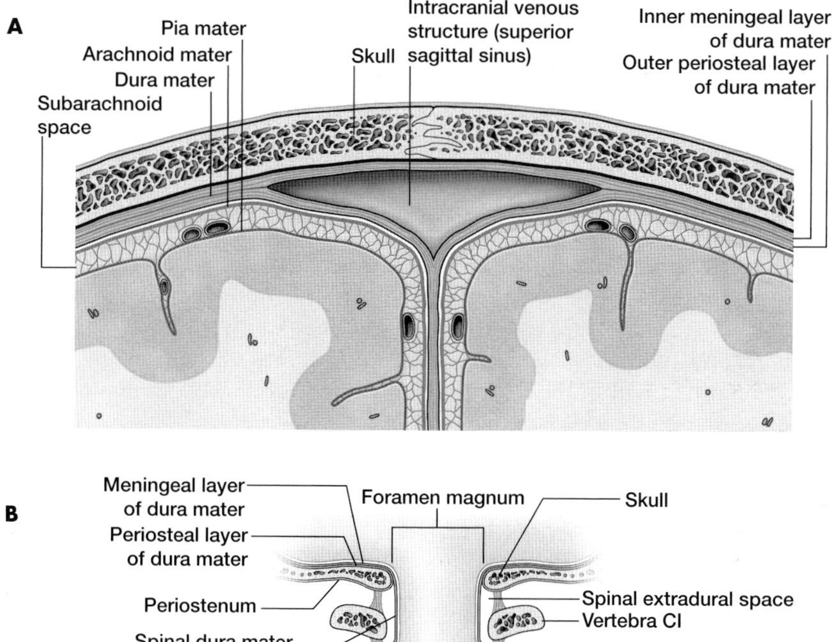

Fig. 2.10 The meninges. (Adapted from Drake et al 2005)

called the dura mater, is dense connective tissue. The middle layer is called the arachnoid mater and is a more delicate layer of fibres that form a web-like membrane. Between the arachnoid mater and the third layer, called the pia mater, is the subarachnoid space through which CSF flows. The pia mater is a very thin membrane that adheres directly to the surface of the brain and spinal cord.

SUMMARY

The CNS comprises the brain and spinal cord. For the purposes of this introduction to basic neuroanatomy, spinal cord structures have not been included as they do not often form a component of neuropsychological observations. Starting at the base of the brain, the brainstem comprises the medulla, pons, reticular formation and cerebellum.

The medulla forms a continuation of the spinal cord and contains all the ascending and descending fibre tracts interconnecting the brain and the spinal cord. A majority of the cranial nerves enter and leave the brain from the medulla and its functions include a role in respiration, heart action, gastrointestinal function and blood pressure.

The pons is located superior to the medulla. It contains both ascending and descending fibre tracts and plays a role in controlling respiration, blood pressure and heart rhythms, as well as contributing to feeding behaviour and facial expression. At the core of the brainstem lies the reticular formation which plays a role in muscle tone, postural reflexes, the preparation of the cortex for the arrival of sensory input, and arousal.

Posterior to the medulla and pons is the cerebellum. It is primarily concerned with the regulation of motor coordination, fines tunes motor activity and plays a role in the learning of skilled movements.

The midbrain is the most anterior portion of the brainstem that maintains the basic tubular structure of the spinal cord. It contains nuclei important to the visual and auditory systems and the cranial nerves that control eye movement. Contained within the midbrain is a nucleus of darkly pigmented cells, the substantia nigra, which is involved in movement.

Next we move into the territory of the major subcortical systems. The thalamus is located at the top of the brainstem and functions as a relay point for the major sensory systems projecting to the cerebral cortex. The thalamus plays a role in pain sensation, attention and alertness. The hypothalamus lies inferior to the thalamus and secretes hormones that control the pituitary glands, which are responsible for physical growth, fight or flight reactions, sexual responses and many other physical expressions of mental states.

The hippocampus (meaning sea horse), a small curved brain structure, is situated between the corpus callosum and temporal lobe. As part of the limbic system, it is involved in the learning and memorization processes.

The basal ganglia, meanwhile, surround the thalamus and are enclosed by the cerebral cortex and the cerebral white matter. The basal ganglia form the major part of the extrapyramidal motor system and, as such, are involved in the control of movement.

Lastly, we come to the brain's outermost surface layer, the cerebral cortex, which controls movement, sensory and somatosensory information and is involved in the higher functions and cognition.

Blood is supplied to the brain by way of the internal carotid artery and the vertebral artery; it is protected from pathogens and toxins by the blood–brain barrier. The ventricular system within the brain produces CSF which serves to: protect the brain from damage, support brain structures, provide a means for the disposal of waste products and provide a medium for the transport of hormones to other areas of the brain.

Finally, the brain is protected by a number of layers of tissue including the scalp, skull and meninges, incorporating the dura mater, arachnoid mater and pia mater.

REFERENCES

Aggleton J P 1992 The amygdala: neurobiological aspects of emotion, memory and mental dysfunction. Wiley, New York

Chozick, B 1986 The behavioural effects of lesions of the amygdala: a review. International Journal of Neuroscience 29:205–221

Crossman A R, Neary D 2000 Neuroanatomy, 2nd edn. Churchill Livingstone, Edinburgh, p 2, 9, 31
Drake R L, Vogl W, Mitchell A W M 2005 Grays Anatomy for Students. Churchill Livingstone, Edinburgh, p 782
Olds J, Milner P 1954 Positive reinforcement produced by electrical stimulation of septal area and other regions of rat brain. Journal of Comparative and Physiological Psychology 47:419–427
Smart T 2001 Human Body. Dorling Kindersley, London
Waugh A, Grant A 2001 Ross and Wilson Anatomy and Physiology in Health and Illness, 9th edn. Churchill Livingstone, Edinburgh, p 49, 100, 148

FURTHER READING

Carpenter M B 1991 Core text of neuroanatomy, 4th edn. Williams & Wilkins, Maryland
Goldberg S 2003 Clinical neuroanatomy made ridiculously simple: interactive edition. Medmaster, Miami
Pinel J P, Edwards M E 1996 A colorful introduction to the anatomy of the human brain: a brain and psychology coloring book. Allyn & Bacon, Boston

Functional neuroanatomy 3

OVERVIEW

Now that we have looked briefly at the structure of the brain, we will examine more closely the structure, connections and functions linked with each of the lobes of the cortex and the disorders that can arise as a result of damage in these areas.

During its evolution, different regions of the brain have become specialized to perform different tasks. As a result, three types of cortex have been identified with regard to the general functions that they serve. These are the motor, sensory, and association cortices.

Motor cortex projects to the motor systems and sensory cortex to the sensory systems. Fundamentally, however, only a small proportion of the cerebral cortex as a whole is given over to these basic sensory and motor processes. The remainder is known as association cortex and it is within this area that the highest functions take place. Thus, the association cortex has direct connections to neither the sensory nor motor systems, but is involved in the complex processing of information from multiple inputs.

The four primary association areas of the brain are located in the frontal, temporal, parietal and occipital lobes, and it is these areas that we tend to think of when making any sort of foray into the neuropsychological realm as they appear to underpin that which we classify as distinctly human; for example personality, language and emotion. It is to these four areas, then, that we will confine ourselves while looking at the main brain functions and dysfunctions. However, as stated in the previous chapter, while the localization of function has its uses, it also has its limitations, and while it is tempting to isolate a particular function to a specific area of the brain, we must remember that when dealing with a system as intricate and complex as the brain, what you see may not necessarily be what you get.

COGNITIVE FUNCTIONS

Generally speaking, and with the previous caution in mind, cognitive functions can be conceptualized as either localized or distributed. Localized functions are thought of as being lateralized to one hemisphere and often only one part of a hemisphere. They can also be subdivided into functions associated with either the dominant or non-dominant hemisphere. Distributed functions, on the other hand, are those that are not strictly localized to one single, lateralized area of the brain. Impairment of these functions, therefore, does not typically arise from localized damage to the tissues but from comparatively extensive and usually bilateral damage.

With regard to localized functions, we generally think of language, the prosodic components of language, praxis, calculation, and complex visuoperceptual and visuospatial skills as being localized within a hemisphere of the brain. In terms of the distributed functions, disturbances of attention, memory, personality, and emotion are frequently encountered, reflecting the reliance of these functions on multiple distributed portions of the brain tissue and the connections between these.

We will, of course, be looking at the anatomical representations of these functions in more detail later on. In the meantime, however, it may be useful to provide a brief discussion of the normal workings of at least some of these systems and the nomenclature associated with them.

Attention

Impairments of attention are amongst the most commonly seen. In contrast to the neuropsychological deficits than can result from more localized damage to the brain, disorders of attention very often occur following injuries to a variety of different cortical and subcortical systems as well as from non-specific physiological factors that affect arousal and metabolic state. Attention, therefore, can be thought of as being a distributed function.

Attention consists of a set of active processes that influence the interface between other cognitive functions such as perception and memory. Attention, therefore, allows us to select important sensory information for further processing and increase or decrease our use of other cognitive processes.

The components of attention, then, include sensory selection, through which sensory input is selected for additional cognitive processing; response selection and control, which allow allocation of attentional resources for response selection and the control of our behavioural responses; attentional capacity and control, which govern the degree of focus we give to a task; automatic and controlled processing, governing our responses to a given stimulus; and sustained attention, which represents the maintenance of optimal performance over the time required to complete a given task.

Our level of arousal and our energy reserves are important factors in our attentional performance. If, then, we experience high levels of fatigue, the consequent effect on attention will be observed in not only tasks requiring attentional skills but also in its impact on other cognitive functions reliant on attention.

Memory

Clearly, any life form capable of retaining information from past experience is at an advantage when similar events occur again. It is for this reason that almost all organisms have some rudimentary form of memory, where new information is gathered by the sensory systems, processed by cortical systems that provide meaning and make associations, and stored for later use.

In human beings, memory is thought to involve: the gathering of information perceived by the senses; the brief cortical storage and processing of this information in a system known as working memory; the movement of this processed material to subcortical structures for further processing; and movement from these subcortical structures for storage throughout widely distributed areas of the cortex. Being reliant on a number of cortical and subcortical structures, memory is thought of, again, as a distributed cognitive function. Furthermore, it can be subdivided into a number of different areas.

Declarative or explicit memories are those that we can consciously bring to mind. Such storage involves episodic memory, the recollection of events that have occurred in the past (for example recalling having breakfast in the morning), and semantic memory, the recollection of facts (for example that an egg has an oval shape).

Procedural or implicit memory, conversely, is that which is retained as learned skill, such as a repetitive motor response or cognitive operation, and usually brought into conscious processing. For example, the motor operations required to learn how to drive a car can be difficult to master but become unconscious with repeated use. Procedural memories include skills learning, priming, simple classical conditioning, operant conditioning and habituation.

Memory can also be categorized by its temporal characteristics. To illustrate: working or short-term memory involves very brief storage of information while it is being interpreted, while long-term memory stores information for much longer periods of time.

Language

Language is mediated mostly by regions of the left cerebral hemisphere. These include Broca's area in the frontal lobe, which stores the motor programmes directing the movement and coordination of speech, and Wernicke's area in the temporal lobe, which provides the conversion of auditory input into meaningful information. Language, therefore, is thought of as localized cognitive function.

Wernicke's and Broca's areas are additionally connected to each other by way of a pathway that helps to mediate the expression of language in speech. Wernicke's area is also connected to the primary sensory areas by functional pathways. Such connections mediate incoming information in different sensory modalities. For example, the pathway between the primary visual area and Wernicke's area mediates reading while the pathway to the somatosensory area mediates tactile language comprehension, such as that needed for Braille reading.

Early in the investigation of laterality and language, it was discovered that, in the majority of people, the left cerebral hemisphere was primarily responsible for the control of speech, with the right hemisphere playing only a minor part in the language process. However, later research has indicated that the right hemisphere is capable of more than was originally thought.

Briefly, while the right hemisphere has little articulatory capacity, it has been found to play an important role in other aspects of language. Essentially, the right hemisphere's role in language comprehension is to extract meaning from linguistic material. This contribution to language processing falls into two main areas: prosody and inference.

In the right hemisphere, the regions equivalent to Broca's and Wernicke's areas in the left hemisphere are responsible for the tonal quality of speech output and the tonal comprehension of information. To give an example of the prosodic components of speech output, an experiment is to utter the words 'what is this thing called love' with different inflections providing different meanings to the listener. For instance, one might say the sentence with a rising inflection at the end to indicate that it is a question: 'What is this thing called love?' Alternatively, one might place the rising inflection in another portion of the sentence to give another, subtly different meaning: 'What is this thing called? . . . Love.'

In addition, determining the theme of a story can help in interpreting ambiguous information. For instance, making inferences about what has not been explicitly stated, and anticipating what information will be presented next helps us to gather important information. A good example of a linguistic form that is designed to undermine this system is the joke.

A joke is funny because it is usually constructed in a manner whereby it forms a coherent story but the punch-line contains a surprise or twist that, nevertheless, coheres with the rest of the story. Damage to the areas of the right hemisphere involved in inference from narrative produces an inability to comprehend a coherent theme in stories, which results in difficulty in comprehending jokes. Right hemisphere damage, then, produces difficulties with following the thread of a story, making inferences about what is being said, and the interpretation of non-literal aspects of language such as metaphors and indirect requests.

THE FRONTAL LOBES

Once the target area for possibly the most notorious of all psychosurgical procedures, the prefrontal lobotomy, the frontal lobes are, perhaps, the most difficult to both describe and conceptualize neuropsychologically. This, no doubt, arises from the complex nature of the functions associated with the frontal areas (Luria 1973) and the quality of the dysfunctions that result from damage in this region. It is here, then, as with no other area, that damage can cause such a wide variety of symptoms (Kolb & Whishaw 1996).

Evolutionarily, the frontal lobes are the most recent development in our species and are the last to fully mature in individuals. Anatomically, they are the most anterior and largest of the brain's lobes, making up approximately one-third of the cerebral cortex, which perhaps accounts for their vulnerability to injury, with magnetic resonance imaging (MRI) studies having shown that the frontal area is the most common region of injury following mild-to-moderate traumatic brain injury (Levin et al 1987).

The frontal lobes are divided from the temporal lobe by the Sylvian fissure and the parietal lobe by the central fissure (Fig. 3.1) and can be further sub-

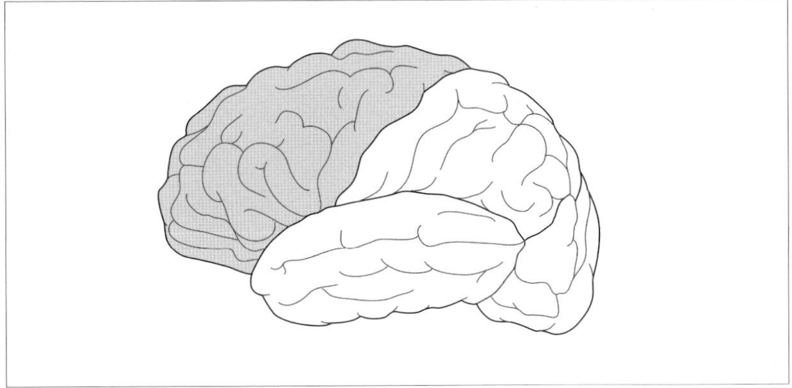

Fig. 3.1 The frontal lobe.

divided into the primary motor region, the premotor region and the prefrontal region, which differ from each other functionally. Importantly, the frontal regions do not receive primary sensory information but they have afferent connections with other visual, auditory, and somatosensory regions within the brain and a number of complex projections from various subcortical structures (Powell & Wilson 1994).

As such, therefore, the frontal lobes play a fundamental role in acting as an 'executive' in the control of other systems, contributing significantly to complex brain–behaviour relationships and helping to define what we classify as unique to us, as both members of a particular species and as individuals (Guilmette 1997).

To illustrate the complexity of this relationship: it is often the case that patients with extensive injury to the frontal lobes will demonstrate distinct changes in their behaviour, emotions and personality, while conversely demonstrating little decrement on tests of intellect (Banich 1997). This is because the impairment often associated with frontal lobe damage frequently involves abilities that are not measured by conventional intellectual measures, which tend to assess well-established skills and old learning rather than the ability to solve new problems or exercise judgement (Lezak 1995).

Thus, in simple terms, while the frontal lobes appear to play a complex role in our whole behavioural repertoire, through a contribution to motor function, olfaction, language, attention, memory, problem solving, abstract reasoning, impulse control, emotion, personality, and environmental, social and sexual behaviour, they are not easily amenable to assessment in terms of quantitative evaluation. With this important point in mind, then, what can we usefully articulate with regard to specific frontal lobe functioning?

Much of our knowledge with regard to neuropsychological functioning has come not only from our observations of the fully functional brain but from the consequences of damage to particular regions. To illustrate these complex and multifaceted functions, then, it will probably be most useful to look at the variety of disorders that can occur with injury to the frontal lobes and their various functional divisions.

The primary and premotor divisions

Motor function

The most posterior of the main divisions of the frontal lobe is located just anterior to the central sulcus. The primary motor cortex, sometimes called the motor strip, implements movement actions generated by the adjacent premotor cortex and is, therefore, responsible for the mediation of movement.

As is the case with somatosensory functions, which we will look at later, the body is representatively but inversely mapped onto this motor tissue. It is also distorted by the amount of tissue given over to a motor function. For example, the area representative of vocal cords, a relatively small anatomical unit, is much larger than that given over to the shoulder or trunk. We can conclude, therefore, that this disproportionate distortion is based on the level of fine motor control undertaken in the particular body part and not its relative size.

This division also has important connections with the cerebellum, basal ganglia and the thalamus, and lesions in this area result in reduced speed and accuracy of movement as well as weakness or paralysis in the contralateral side of the body.

The premotor or secondary motor area, lying anterior to the primary motor area, generates motor programmes that are relayed to the primary motor cortex and integrates motor skills and learned action sequences (Damasio & Anderson 1993). Lesions in this area will tend to cause apraxia or dyspraxia, a disintegration of the components of complex motor actions producing dyscoordination.

The prefrontal division

Lesions of the most anterior portions of the frontal lobes, the prefrontal regions, can have serious consequences in terms of both cognitive and affective functioning in a variety of ways that are of particular interest to neuropsychologists.

Olfaction

Olfaction is commonly impaired with damage to the orbitofrontal cortex, while bilateral lesions to the orbitofrontal and mesial cortex can produce anosmia, an inability to detect odours at either nostril (Eslinger et al 1982).

Attention

The prefrontal cortex is one of the many structures involved in attentional functioning and the frontal lobes appear to play a significant role in the direction and regulation of attention. Thus, patients with frontal lobe damage appear to be slow to react to stimuli and have poor attentional focus (Stuss 1993), and have both poor concentration and high distractibility (Janowsky et al 1989).

Memory

The dorsolateral prefrontal cortex appears to be significantly involved in working memory, the temporary store for information necessary for the completion of complex cognitive tasks such as comprehension, learning or problem solving. Working memory represents the first stage in short-term memory processes and is highly important in terms of executive functions, which we will look at later.

Lezak (1995) refers to a form of frontal amnesia as 'not remembering to remember', which appears to be the result of a lack of drive to recall rather than a mnestic disorder per se, as typically, such problems do not register as specific memory deficits on neuropsychological testing. Thus patients commonly appear to demonstrate disturbances of everyday memory, for example misplacing keys (Selby 2000).

Damage to the prefrontal cortex, however, also produces a number of other memory problems including difficulties in the ability to organize, search and query prospective memory (that portion of memory we use for recalling future events); for example forthcoming appointments (Shimamura 1990). This, in turn, can lead to temporal memory failures, errors in the ability to sequence events in their correct temporal order (Milner et al 1991) and source memory failures, recollecting the source of information (Janowsky et al 1989). To say nothing of the frontal lobe patient's susceptibility to interference (Benson 1993), which itself has a profound effect on memory.

Language

With respect to language functioning, the left frontal lobe appears to play an important role in the processing of language whilst other frontal areas play a role in the tonal quality and motor expression of speech.

Amongst the most widely known deficits to occur with frontal damage is Broca's aphasia (also known as non-fluent or expressive aphasia) ranging from complete mutism to non-fluent, agrammatical speech produced as single words or phrases with poor inflection and intonation, and poor naming skills. Very often written language expression follows a similar pattern.

Executive functions

The so-called executive functions of the frontal lobes are a broad set of abilities necessary for the planning, organization, direction and control of behaviour crucial to independent functioning (Guilmette 1997). They are the complex processes by which an individual goes about performing a novel problem-solving task from its inception to completion (Sbordone 2000) and include: the formulation of goals and the consequences of these, the generation of response alternatives, the choice and initiation of goal-directed behaviour, self-monitoring, the correction and modification of behaviour, and persistence (Malloy et al 1998).

Typically, this spectrum of self-regulatory behavioural functions is associated with the frontal lobes. However, they probably require the input of a number of other brain regions to operate correctly and while there is no specific definition of the skills that fall under this heading, they have been broadly categorized into a number of different functional areas. Lezak (1995) has grouped these functions into four distinct components: volition, planning, purposive action and effective performance. Box 3.1 shows a number of the observable deficits lying in each of these component areas.

Personality and social functioning

One of the most striking changes often observed with damage to the frontal lobes is an alteration in personality and social behaviour. Perhaps the most well-known example of this is the case of Phineas Gage (Harlow 1868). Gage, an explosives worker, survived a blast that drove a metre-long tamping iron up through his cheek and into the front of his head, damaging the left frontal lobe. He made a good physical recovery and, contrary to what might be expected, many of his cognitive skills remained intact. However, his personality appeared to have changed. He became profane, irreverent, capricious, and impatient. He lost his sense of responsibility and appeared to have no difficulties in disregarding social rules.

At the time of Gage's death in 1861, very little neuropsychological interest was shown in these observations. However, as the discipline of psychiatry progressed in the 20th Century, more and more studies of the effects of lesions in the frontal lobes on personality concluded that damage in the orbital regions of the prefrontal cortex produced more dramatic changes than did dorsolateral lesions (Kolb & Whishaw 1996).

In 1975, Blumer & Benson took this observation further and described two specific types of personality change observed in patients with damage to the frontal lobes: pseudodepressive and pseudopsychopathic. Patients with pseu-

Box 3.1 Deficits observed in executive function areas

(Adapted from Sbordone 2000)

Volition
Loss of social awareness
Loss of motivation
Loss of interests
Indifference
Apathy
Poor awareness of cognitive or behavioural problems
Need for external structure

Planning
Loss of abstraction and conceptual reasoning
Inflexible thinking
Poor planning and organization
Disorganized thinking
Disorganized behaviour
Socially inappropriate behaviour

Purposive action
Distractibility
Loss of initiative
Difficulties in simultaneous processing
Emotional lability
Impatience
Difficulty in performing novel tasks
Difficulty in maintaining response set
Tangential thinking

Effective performance
Perseveration
Poor ability to identify or correct errors
Poor ability to complete tasks
Poor problem solving
Poor use of planning or strategies

dodepressive personality change usually have damage to the dorsal frontal regions and are characterized as lacking in drive, spontaneity, motivation and interest. They are observed as apathetic and indifferent, with little verbal or emotional output and reduced sexual interest. Patients with pseudopsychopathic personality change, on the other hand, usually have damage to the orbitofrontal regions and are characterized as impulsive, impatient, and immature. They lack tact or restraint, have increased motor activity, display difficulties with social awareness, use crude language, and exhibit promiscuous sexual behaviour.

It has also been observed that, while many of these symptoms can be seen in the greater number of patients with frontal lobe damage, with the full spectrum probably only exhibited by patients with bilateral involvement, there is a tendency toward pseudodepression with lesions to the left frontal lobe and a tendency toward pseudopsychopathy with lesions to the right frontal lobe.

With these changes in mind, then, it is easy to see, as in the case of pseudodepression where there is a degree of inertia, apathy and indifference, the lure of the prefrontal lobotomy as a form of treatment in the late 1940s and early 1950s prior to the availability of antipsychotic and antidepressive drugs. Thankfully, however, the procedure is now extremely rare (Tippin & Henn 1982).

Other conditions associated with frontal lobe damage

Environmental dependency is a syndrome in which the patient responds to the stimuli in the environment in a habitual manner without regard to the appropriateness or necessity of the behaviour (Hoffman & Bill 1992). An example would be the patient who, upon seeing plates in a kitchen, would begin to wash them whether the plates needed to be washed or not.

Utilization behaviour is similar to environmental dependency and refers to the patient's use of objects in the environment without a specific goal; for example sipping from an empty cup (Lhermitte 1983). Two types of this disorder have been identified (Shallice et al 1989). 'Incidental' behaviour occurs when the patient uses objects nearby in the environment when performing a task and 'induced' utilization behaviour occurs when the patient observes a cue in the manner of others in the environment that appears to prompt the use of objects.

'Alien hand' or intermanual conflict can occur with lesions to the motor areas and corpus callosum producing a condition whereby the patient's left hand often acts as if it were independently motivated and the patient feels they have no control over the hand's movements (Goldberg & Bloom 1990).

Perseveration refers to the continuation of an activity, either motor or cognitive, after it is appropriate. It reflects an inability to shift responses or stop responding after the termination of the causative stimulus (Guilmette 1997). The patient with frontal lobe damage might, therefore, find it difficult, if not impossible, to stop behaving in a certain manner.

Confabulation is sometimes seen in patients with extensive damage to the frontal lobes and is most common among patients with an additional impairment of memory ability. The term describes a tendency to manufacture impulsive answers to questions, with responses sometimes being somewhat far-fetched and imaginative.

Reduplication syndrome is similar to confabulation and involves the patient confabulating that the current environment is actually another place that is similar to the current setting but has a different name and location; for example the patient may claim that the current setting, usually a hospital, is their home. Typically, the confabulated location is geographically elsewhere and familiar to the patient. Moreover, the patient will usually maintain this confabulation even when confronted with contradictory information.

For a brief summary of frontal lobe functions please refer also to Box 3.2.

THE TEMPORAL LOBES

Lying posterior to the frontal lobe, inferior to the parietal lobe and anterior to the occipital lobe, the temporal lobe structures (Fig. 3.2) mediate a number of functions including: auditory processing, language comprehension, memory, olfaction and the emotions. Also, one-half of the visual projections pass through the temporal lobe as they make their way from the eyes to the primary visual cortex in the occipital lobe.

Olfaction

The olfactory system does not have the extensive cortical representation that vision, audition, and tactile sensations do in the cortex (Kolb & Whishaw 1996). However, despite the fact that the olfactory bulbs (the primary sense organs for olfaction) are located beneath the frontal lobe and the primary olfactory cortex is located in the orbitofrontal region of the frontal lobe, odour

Box 3.2 A summary of frontal lobe functions

Main divisions

Primary motor
Implementation of movement programmes from premotor cortex

Premotor
Selection and direction of movements

Prefrontal
Control of cognitive processes

Prefrontal cortex functions

Selection of behaviour based on short-term memory
Attention span
Perseverance
Planning
Judgement
Impulse control
Organization
Self-monitoring
Problem solving
Learning from experience
Ability to experience and express emotions
Empathy

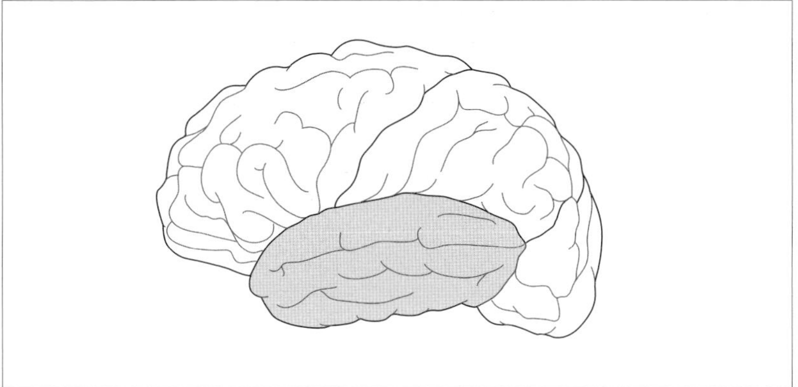

Fig. 3.2 The temporal lobe.

perception appears to require intact temporal lobes (Eskenazi et al 1986) and is particularly vulnerable to damage in the right temporal lobe where lesions to the right temporal and orbitofrontal cortex have been associated with deficits in odour recognition memory (Jones-Gotman & Zatorre 1993).

Audition

The temporal lobes are particularly important for audition because they contain both the primary auditory cortex and the auditory association areas and it is these areas in which activity increases during processing which requires auditory attention. Thus, bilateral damage or damage to both temporal lobes may result in cortical deafness; that is, deafness arising from damage to the primary cortical areas responsible for audition rather than dysfunction of other parts of the auditory system, for example the tympanic membranes (ear drums) or the auditory ossicles (the bones of hearing in the middle ear that transmit the vibrations of the ear drum to the inner ear). On the other hand, less severe, unilateral damage (damage to the temporal lobe in a single hemisphere of the brain) can lead to reduction in auditory acuity rather than complete deafness.

Lesions to other areas of the auditory cortex can also produce a number of other deficits, such as the loss of musical comprehension for pitch, tone, harmony, rhythm, or melody, known as sensory amusia and the inability to comprehend non-verbal sounds, known as auditory agnosia for non-speech sounds.

Vision

In addition to auditory functions, the temporal lobes play an important role in visual processing and visual item recognition, and contain portions of the visual projections as they pass to the primary visual cortex in the occipital lobe. Thus, damage to the underlying visual projections can produce a contralateral upper homonymous hemianopia, a visual field defect affecting the upper quadrants of the visual field (Lindsay et al 1997) and a number of visuoperceptual deficits such as difficulties in face recognition (Damasio et al 1982).

Language

In addition to containing the primary auditory cortex, the temporal lobes also play a central role in language reception and comprehension. It is for this reason that damage to the left posterior region of the temporal region results in Wernicke's or receptive aphasia, a disorder characterized by poor comprehension in both written and spoken language (Selby 2000).

Typically, speech in such patients is fluent, with correct grammar and normal tone and prosody. However, while comprehension is impaired there is also usually significant difficulty observed with word finding. There is also the presence of neologisms, or words which have no meaning, and paraphasias, errors of expression that involve either the substitution of a similar sounding word or a word of similar meaning, for example 'rog' for dog or 'knife' for fork.

Memory

Historically, the temporal lobes have been associated with memory. At the cortical level, the temporal lobe is thought to play a role in the triggering of mechanisms for recall (Lezak 1995) and the organization of the components of memory from different locations within the brain to enable systematic and complete recall (Nauta 1964).

Lying beneath the temporal lobes are the limbic system structures, the amygdala and hippocampus, both of which play an important role in the consolidation of new memories. Damage to these areas often produces anterograde amnesia (an inability to consolidate new memories) or retrograde amnesia (an inability to retrieve information from long-term stores).

There also appears to be a dissociation between the type of memory deficit and the side of the brain where damage is observed. To illustrate, it appears that verbal memory deficits are greater if the left temporal lobe is involved (Frisk & Milner 1990) and that non-verbal deficits are greater if the right temporal lobe is involved (Smith & Milner 1981).

Personality and emotion

The temporal lobes, like the frontal lobes, also appear to play a role in personality and the emotions. This is, of course, not surprising given this region's close connections with the limbic system. Once again, a great deal of what we have come to understand about the temporal lobe's contribution to function has come from our observations of dysfunction and damage. However, in this case, perhaps the most abundant source of observations with regard to the temporal lobes and their association with emotion has come from the study of temporal lobe epilepsy (TLE).

We will look at epilepsy in greater detail in a later chapter. At present, however, it is enough to operationally define epilepsy as the abnormal electrical activity of the brain, with TLE being an example of the abnormal electrical activity associated with, and usually originating from, the temporal lobes.

In TLE, certain types of interictal or between seizures behaviour in many sufferers has led to the hypothesis that there may be a temporal lobe or epileptic personality. Bear & Fedio (1977), in a quantitative study of this behaviour, concluded that there were some 18 behavioural features that could be observed. These included: emotionality, mania, depression, guilt, humourlessness, altered sexual interest, aggression, anger and hostility, hypergraphia (excessive writing), religiosity, philosophical interest, a sense of personal destiny, hypermoralism, dependency, paranoia, obsessionalism, circumstantiality, and viscosity.

These observations have been disputed by other researchers and have caused a great deal of controversy, with many feeling that these features could simply represent generalized features of personality change associated with any form of medical or neurological illness. Despite this debate, however, it seems that there is some agreement with regard to generalized behaviour, in that many of these patients tend to be obsessive and over-inclusive in their thinking, often satisfying some or all of the requirements for obsessive-compulsive personality. Their speech and thinking is viscous and ponderous with a tendency towards loquacity and the insistence on the elaboration of fine and often tedious distinctions, with outbursts of irritability (Restak 1995).

Anxiety, anxiety-related disorders and depression also appear to occur more frequently in TLS patients (Koth-Weser et al 1988), as do psychoses (McKenna et al 1985).

Other conditions associated with temporal lobe damage

Kluver-Bucy syndrome is a rare condition resulting from damage to the temporal lobes and amygdala resulting in apathy, passivity, flattened emotional responses, hyperorality (a tendency to examine objects orally), hyperphagia (excessive eating), amnesia, visual agnosia, and hypersexuality. Damage to these temporolimbic structures has also been associated with episodic dyscontrol syndrome (EDS) a disorder of episodic hyperirritability, aggressive outbursts, and the sudden onset of dysphoric mood states.

For a brief summary of temporal lobe functions please refer also to Box 3.3.

THE PARIETAL LOBES

Encircled by the frontal, temporal and occipital lobes, the parietal lobe (Fig. 3.3) is sometimes referred to as the posterior association cortex. The parietal lobes can be divided into two functional regions. The first involves sensation and perception and the second is concerned with the integration of sensory input and primarily with the visual system.

Box 3.3 A summary of temporal lobe functions

Primary functions
Audition
Processing of auditory input
Visual object recognition and categorization
Long-term storage of auditory sensory input
Emotional labelling of sensory input and memories

Dominant side functions (usually left sided)
Perception of words
Processing of language-related sounds
Memory
Visual and auditory processing
Verbal learning

Non-dominant side functions (usually right sided)
Perception of melodies
Perception of facial expression
Processing of vocal intonation
Rhythm
Visual learning

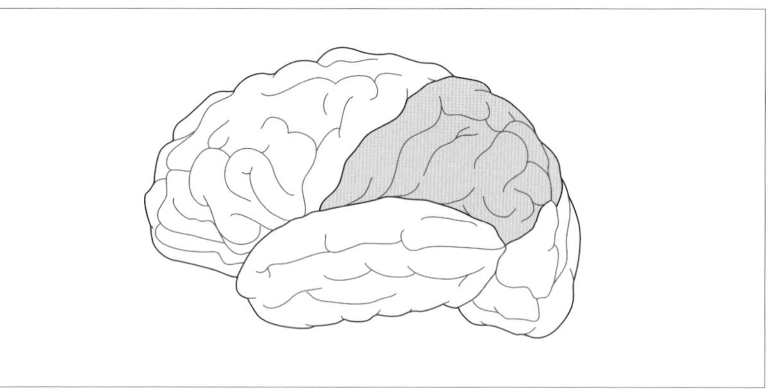

Fig. 3.3 The parietal lobe.

Given its anatomical positioning posterior to the frontal and temporal lobes and anterior to the occipital lobe, it is easy to appreciate this integrative role with the assimilation of information from various sensory modalities (visual, auditory and tactile senses), the combining of information from the internal state with information from the external sensory world, and the integration of memory with sensory experience. Apart from its direct role in somatosensory systems, then, the parietal lobe plays a multimodal, associational function within the brain. Thus, lesions arising from damage in this area can and do produce a wide variety of often confusing deficits of integration between sensory information, memory, and internal representations of the sensory world.

To illustrate, it is here that we process sensations such as the presence of pain, temperature change, pressure sensitivity, touch and body position;

visually guide movement to produce writing or drawing, etc.; process spatial information; and integrate information into other cognitive functions thought to have a spatial component, such as reading or arithmetic.

Sensation

The primary somatosensory cortex is located directly posterior to the central fissure and receives information from bodily receptors concerning tactile stimulation, pain, pressure, temperature and proprioception.

Much like the motor area in the frontal lobe, the body is representatively mapped onto this somatosensory tissue in an inverted manner. That is to say that the body is represented in a roughly bottom to top and left to right reversal in the tissues. This somatosensory map of the body is also distorted by the proportional density of information received and, therefore, by the number of receptors. For example, the area representative of the hands is larger than that for the lower back.

Damage to this area often causes loss of the fine discrimination of touch on the contralateral side of the body. Thus, there is often a reduction in the sensitivity of touch, for example a poor ability to discriminate between two different textures; a reduction in the threshold for frequency of stimulation, for example difficulty in determining the number of times the hand is touched in rapid succession; and a reduction in two point discrimination, the ability to discern two points of touch as these points are brought closer and closer together.

Integration

The second function of the parietal lobes is to construct an internal spatial coordinate system that represents the world around us. Thus, patients with damage to the more posterior portions of the parietal lobes often show striking deficits, such as abnormalities in body image and spatial relations (Kandel et al 1991).

The left parietal cortex integrates visual perception with the motor processes needed to reproduce drawings, write or perform mathematical calculations, while the right contributes more significantly to visuospatial skills such as map reading (Selby 2000). Damage to the left or right parietal lobes, therefore, results in a number of specific symptoms where other functions are integrated to form a more complex whole. Boxes 3.4 and 3.5 list a number of the disorders arising from left or right parietal lobe damage.

Other conditions associated with parietal lobe damage

Gerstmann's syndrome is a constellation of symptoms thought to occur following damage to the left parietal lobe. It is characterized by a left/right confusion, finger agnosia, agraphia and acalculia. Since their first identification by Gerstmann in 1924, however, there has been some debate as to whether or not these symptoms can be grouped together to localize damage within the brain.

Box 3.4 Disorders associated with left parietal lobe damage

Disorder	*Symptoms*
Aphasia	Poor comprehension Echolalia Jargon speech Poor awareness of the language disability
Constructional apraxia	Inability to copy visually presented stimuli
Ideomotor apraxia	Inability to copy movements or make gestures to command
Acalculia	Inability to perform mathematical computations
Agraphia	An inability to write; usually observed as a function of aphasia
Finger agnosia	An inability to recognize the fingers on either hand
Left/right disorientation	Inability to discern left from right

Box 3.5 Disorders associated with right parietal lobe damage

Disorder	*Symptoms*
Contralateral neglect	A disorder of spatial attention causing a failure to attend to stimuli (visual, auditory or tactile) presented on the neglected side of the body
Constructional apraxia	Inability to copy with visually presented stimuli
Dyscalculia	Difficulty in performing mathematical operations based on spatial relationships, e.g. using decimal places
Dressing apraxia	A spatial disorientation characterized by an inability to organize and relate body parts to clothing
Topographic disturbance	Disruption of the internal spatial representation of the external environment
Anosagnosia	The denial or loss of recognition of physical disability

Asomatognosia usually occurs as a result of damage to the more anterior portions of the parietal lobes and represents a loss of knowledge or sense of one's own body or bodily condition (Kolb & Whishaw 1996). It includes a number of most curious conditions that, because of their nature, are often mistaken for psychological or emotional reactions to illness.

Anosagnosia, for example, is a biological loss of insight into illness occurring most commonly with damage to the right parietal region and is often accompanied by hemiplegia, neglect and impaired constructional ability. Anosodiaphoria, on the other hand, is a condition where awareness of the illness is intact but there is an indifference to it. Both of these conditions, of course, pose a great challenge in terms of the rehabilitation process, for if the patient is unaware of a particular problem, engagement in treatment may be extremely difficult.

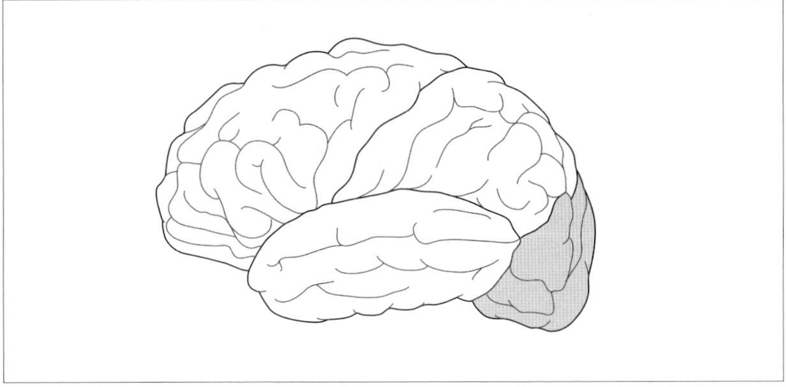

Fig. 3.4 The occipital lobe.

Box 3.6 A summary of parietal lobe functions

Processing of somatosensory input
Bodily awareness
Sensory discrimination
Sensory integration
Spatial orientation
Spatial processing
Visuospatial processing
Visual attention
Visual guidance of movement
Kinaesthesis
Mathematical reasoning

For a brief summary of parietal lobe functions please refer also to Box 3.6.

OCCIPITAL LOBES

Finally, we come to the most posterior of the lobes of the brain (Fig. 3.4), the occipital lobe, the location of the primary visual cortex or, as it is sometimes called, the striate cortex (because of its striped appearance). The occipital lobes form the posterior pole of the cerebral hemispheres. However, the occipital lobes, more than any other, demonstrate the essential imposition of our structural framework on cortical tissue which, generally speaking, has no well-differentiated geographical boundaries.

Thus, there are no specific topographical landmarks to help us differentiate from either the parietal or temporal lobes and this, indeed, has led to some degree of confusion over exact boundaries. Therefore, even though vision is an exclusive function of this area, it should be noted that other visual functions and visual integration also take place in other areas.

Notwithstanding this qualification, then, the primary function of the occipital lobes, as already stated, is visual processing with various subdivisions within the tissues being responsible for form, colour and pattern perception as well as the location of visual stimuli in space.

Vision

Destruction of any part of the visual cortex produces a corresponding loss of vision in part of the visual field, with isolated lesions producing discrete blind spots that, although present, do not hinder the comprehension of visual stimuli. Such areas of loss are known as scotomas. If a greater area of damage occurs but is limited to only the dorsal or ventral portions of the occipital lobe in a single hemisphere, a contralateral quadrant of the visual field is lost. This is known as quadrantonopsia. If, however, the entire occipital cortex of one hemisphere is damaged, then there is a consequent loss of the entire contralateral visual field. This condition is termed hemianopia.

With greater bilateral damage to the visual cortex comes the condition known as cortical blindness where the cortex is unable to process visual information despite the intactness of the optic nerves and retina, and the whole visual field is lost. Incomplete syndromes of cortical blindness are many and varied.

Disorders of higher visual processing involve damage to the visual association cortex and while the visual fields may appear to be normal, the patient will demonstrate an inability to perceive visual objects normally. Such conditions include achromatopsia, which is an inability to perceive colour; motion blindness, a disturbance of the ability to perceive moving objects; and visual agnosia, an inability to recognize visual stimuli.

Visual agnosia falls into two main types. Aperceptive visual agnosia represents a malfunction in the ability to recognize objects when the basic visual functions appear to be intact. Thus, there is a failure to form an overall percept of the object or objects and the patient is unable to describe the whole whilst being able to recognize individual elements of the whole. Associative visual agnosia, on the other hand, refers to an inability to recognize an object although perception of the whole appears to be unaffected.

Other conditions associated with occipital lobe damage

Balint's syndrome, a visual attention and motor disorder, results from bilateral injury to both parietal lobes. It is characterized by an inability to voluntarily control gaze, known as ocular apraxia, an inability to integrate the different components of a visual stimulus, known as simultanagnosia, and the poor ability to accurately reach for an object with visual guidance, known as optic ataxia (Westmoreland 1994).

Patients with Balint's syndrome appear to neglect the peripheral parts of the visual fields and have great difficulty integrating the information from all parts of the visual fields into a useful whole. To illustrate, when shown a picture, the patient may only describe numerous individual details but not recognize the pictured events as a whole. Meanwhile, the optic ataxia associated with this syndrome is manifest as a difficulty in judging distances in visual space and correctly coordinating motor actions based on spatial

Box 3.7 A summary of occipital lobe functions

Primary visual processing	Primary visual association
Localization	Visual interpretation
Form	Visual recognition
Colour	
Pattern	

arrangement. For example, when asked to pour water from a jug into a glass, the patient will miss the glass.

Anton's syndrome, sometimes observed in cases of acute cortical blindness, is a condition whereby patients may deny their blindness and act in a manner that would suggest they are sighted. For example, patients may walk around, bumping into objects and injuring themselves. Anton's syndrome is caused by damage to the occipital lobe which extends from the primary visual cortex into the visual association areas.

Prosopagnosia, a form of visual agnosia, describes the inability to recognize faces (Geschwind 1979). Patients with this disorder may not even be able to recognize their own face in a mirror or photograph (Kolb & Whishaw 1996) and often demonstrate other conditions such as achromatopsia and topographic disturbances.

Alexia, the inability to read, can occur in a number of different forms. However, pure alexia refers to the presence of a reading impairment without a coexisting aphasia or agraphia. Patients with this disorder, therefore, appear to have no disturbance of expressive or receptive language functions and can also write normally, although they frequently cannot read what they have written (Beeson & Rapcsak 1998).

Visual hallucinations, once again, fall into different forms. Simple hallucinations range from flashes of light to complex geometric patterns and can often be observed in patients with migraine involving ischaemia of the occipital lobes (Capruso et al 1998), while complex hallucinations (Kolmel 1985) can form quite remarkably intricate representations of, most commonly, animals or people.

For a brief summary of temporal lobe functions please refer also to Box 3.7.

SUMMARY

The brain may be divided into three types of cortical tissue: motor, sensory, and association cortex. Motor systems and sensory cortex, however, make up only a small proportion of the whole. By far the greatest quantity of tissue resides in the association cortex and it is here that the highest functions take place. The four main areas of the brain associated with these functions are the frontal, temporal, parietal and occipital lobes.

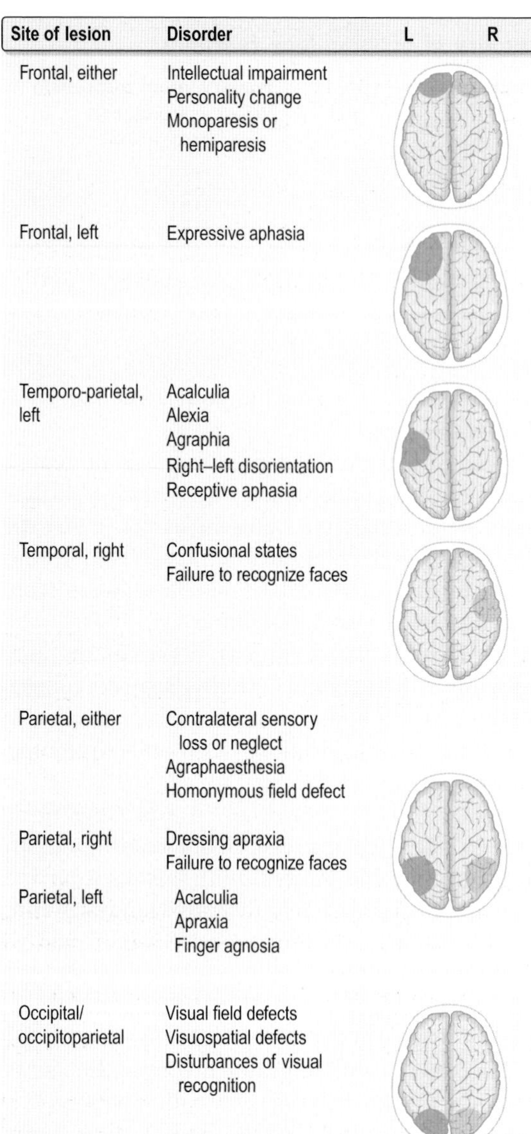

Site of lesion	Disorder	L R
Frontal, either	Intellectual impairment Personality change Monoparesis or hemiparesis	
Frontal, left	Expressive aphasia	
Temporo-parietal, left	Acalculia Alexia Agraphia Right–left disorientation Receptive aphasia	
Temporal, right	Confusional states Failure to recognize faces	
Parietal, either	Contralateral sensory loss or neglect Agraphaesthesia Homonymous field defect	
Parietal, right	Dressing apraxia Failure to recognize faces	
Parietal, left	Acalculia Apraxia Finger agnosia	
Occipital/ occipitoparietal	Visual field defects Visuospatial defects Disturbances of visual recognition	

Fig. 3.5 Summary of damage by area in a right-handed individual. (Adapted from Kumar & Clark 2005)

The frontal lobe is the most anterior portion of the brain. It governs motor function, expressive language and plays a role in memory; it serves to initiate activity and determines how we respond to our environment. It is this lobe we associate strongly with personality and here that we make judgements and control our emotional responses.

The temporal lobe is located posterior to the frontal lobe, inferior to the parietal lobe and anterior to the occipital lobe. It plays a role in audition, language comprehension, visual and verbal memory, vision, olfaction, emotional functioning and, to some degree, personality.

The parietal lobe, meanwhile, lies posterior to the frontal lobe, superior to the temporal lobe and anterior to the occipital lobe. It forms, therefore, a junction between these other cortical areas and provides an integration point for information from other systems. It is concerned with the integration, discrimination and processing of sensory data, the combining of this input with information from the temporal and occipital lobes and plays a role in both awareness of body state and the control of movement.

Finally, the occipital lobes are located posterior to the frontal, temporal and parietal lobes. The occipital lobe contains the primary visual cortex and is responsible for vision. Different parts of the cortex process different aspects of visual stimuli, and other visual association areas give meaning to these visual stimuli.

Damage to these areas gives rise to a number of different symptoms or symptom groupings. A brief summary of some of these symptoms can be seen in Figure 3.5.

REFERENCES

Banich M T 1997 Neuropsychology: the neural basis of mental functions. Houghton Mifflin, New York

Bear D M, Fedio P 1977 Quantitative analysis of interictal behaviour in temporal lobe epilepsy. Archives of Neurology 34:454–467

Beeson P M, Rapcsak S Z 1998 The aphasias. In: Snyder P, Nussbaum, P (eds) Clinical neuropsychology: a pocket handbook for assessment. American Psychological Association, Washington DC

Benson D F 1993 Prefrontal abilities. Behavioural Neurology 6:75–81

Blumer D, Benson D F 1975 Personality changes with frontal and temporal lobe lesions. In: Benson D F, Blumer D (eds) Psychiatric aspects of neurologic disease. Grune and Straton, New York

Capruso D X, Hamsher K deS, Benton A L 1998 Clinical evaluation of visual perception and constructional ability. In: Snyder P, Nussbaum P (eds) Clinical neuropsychology: a pocket handbook for assessment. American Psychological Association, Washington DC

Damasio A R, Anderson S W 1993 The frontal lobes. In: Heilman K M, Valenstein E (eds) Clinical neuropsychology, 3rd edn. Oxford University Press, New York

Damasio A R, Damasio H, Van Hoesen G W 1982 Prosopagnosia: anatomical basis and behavioural mechanisms. Neurology 32:331–341

Eskenazi B, Cain W S, Novelly R A et al 1986 Odor perception in temporal lobe epilepsy patients with and without temporal lobectomy. Neuropsychologia 24:553–562

Eslinger P J, Damasio A R, Van Hoesen G W 1982 Olfactory dysfunction in man: anatomical and behavioural aspects. Brain and Cognition 1:259–285

Frisk V, Milner B 1990 The role of the left hippocampal region in the acquisition and retention of story content. Neuropsychologia 28:349–359

Geschwind N 1979 Specializations of the human brain. Scientific American, 241:180–199

Goldberg G, Bloom K K 1990 The alien hand sign: localization, lateralization and recovery. American Journal of Physical Medicine and Rehabilitation 69:228–238

Guilmette T J 1997 Pocket guide to brain injury, cognitive, and neurobehavioral rehabilitation. Singular Publishing Group, San Diego

Harlow J M 1868 Recovery from the passage of an iron bar through the head. Massachusetts Medical Society Publications, 2:327–346

Hoffman M W, Bill P L 1992 The environmental dependency sydrome, imitation behaviour and utilisation behaviour as presenting symptoms of bi-lateral frontal lobe infarction due to moyamoya disease. South African Medical Journal 81:271–273

Janowsky J S, Shimamura A P, Kritchevsky M, Squire L R 1989 Cognitive impairment following frontal lobe damage and its relevance to human amnesia. Behavioural Neuroscience 103:548–560

Jones-Gotman M, Zatorre R J 1993 Odor recognition memory in humans: role of right temporal and orbitofrontal regions. Brain and Cognition 22:182–198

Kandel J, Schwartz J, Jessell T 1991 Principles of neural science, 3rd edn. Elsevier, New York

Koch-Weser M, Garron D C, Gilley D W et al 1988 Prevalence of psychologic disorders after surgical treatment of seizures. Archives of Neurology 45:1308–1311

Kolb B, Whishaw I Q 1996 Fundamentals of human neuropsychology, 4th edn. W H Freeman, New York

Kolmel H W 1985 Complex visual hallucinations in the hemianopic field. Journal of Neurology, Neurosurgery and Psychiatry 48:29–38

Kumar P, Clark M 2005 Clinical Medicine, 6th edn. Elsevier Saunders, Edinburgh, p 1177

Levin H S, Amparo E, Eisenberg H et al 1987 Magnetic resonance imaging and computerized tomography in relation to the neurobehavioral sequelae of mild and moderate head injuries. Journal of Neurosurgery 66:706–713

Lezak M D 1995 Neuropsychological assessment, 3rd edn. Oxford University Press, Oxford

Lhermitte F 1983 Utilization behaviour and its relation to lesions of the frontal lobes. Brain 106:237–255

Lindsay K W, Bone I, Callander R 1997 Neurology and neurosurgery illustrated, 3rd edn. Churchill Livingstone, Edinburgh

Luria A R 1973 The working brain. Penguin, London

McKenna P J, Kane J M, Parrish K 1985 Psychotic syndromes in epilepsy. American Journal of Psychiatry 142:895–904

Malloy P F, Cohen R A, Jenkins M A 1998 Frontal lobe function and dysfunction. In: Snyder P, Nussbaum P (eds) Clinical neuropsychology: a pocket handbook for assessment. American Psychological Association, Washington DC

Milner B, Corsi P, Leonard G 1991 Frontal lobe contribution to recency judgements. Neuropsychology 29:601–618

Nauta W J 1964 Some brain structures and functions related to memory. Neurosciences Research Progress Bulletin 2(5):1–20

Powell G E, Wilson B A 1994 Introduction to neuropsychology and neuropsychological assessment. In: Lindsay S, Powell G A (eds) Handbook of clinical adult psychology, 2nd edn. Routledge, London

Restak R 1995 Complex partial seizures present diagnostic challenge. Psychiatric Times 12(9)

Sbordone R J 2000 Executive functions of the brain. In: Groth-Marnet G (ed) Neuropsychological assessment in clinical practice: a guide to test interpretation and integration. Wiley, New York

Selby M J 2000 Overview of neurology. In: Groth-Marnet G (ed) Neuropsychological assessment in clinical practice: a guide to test interpretation and integration. Wiley, New York

Shallice T, Burgess P W, Baxter D M et al 1989 The origins of utilisation behaviour. Brain 112:1587–1598

Shimamara A 1990 Aging and memory disorders: a neuropsychological analysis. In: Howe M L, Stones M J, Brainerd C J (eds) Cognitive and behavioural performance factors in atypical aging. Springer-Verlag, New York

Smith M L, Milner B 1981 The role of the right hippocampus in the recall of spatial location. Neuropsychologia 19:781–793

Stuss D T 1993 Assessment of neuropsychological dysfunction in frontal lobe degeneration. Dementia 4:220–225

Tippin J, Henn F A 1982 Modified leukotomy in the treatment of obessional neurosis. American Journal of Psychiatry 139:1601–1603

Westmoreland B F 1994 Medical neurosciences: an approach to anatomy, pathology, and physiology by systems and levels. Little Brown, Boston

FURTHER READING

Filley C M 2002 Neurobehavioral anatomy. Colorado University Press, Boulder
Nolte J 2002 The human brain: an introduction to its functional neuroanatomy, 5th edn. Mosby, St. Louis

Neurological investigations

4

OVERVIEW

Before the 1970s and the advent of non-invasive procedures such as computed tomography (CT), the main imaging investigations available to clinicians were electroencephalography (EEG), skull X-ray, and the more uncomfortable and dangerous airencephalography or pneumoencephalography, a now obsolete radiographic investigation involving the introduction of air or another gas into the intracranial spaces through a lumbar puncture.

Since the 1970s, however, invasive procedures such as this have been superseded by the introduction of more sophisticated techniques which not only serve the purpose, along with the older more established investigations, of data collection in the central nervous system (CNS), but the representation of this data in a useful format.

The main techniques for the investigation of possible structural damage are, of course, CT, EEG and magnetic resonance imaging (MRI), but here we will also look at some of the other diagnostic methods used, such as functional imaging and angiography, and both the advantages and disadvantages of each procedure.

However, whilst extremely valuable in clinical practice, we must also keep in mind the very important thought that, while these various procedures have revolutionized the way in which we view the brain, they are by no means perfect and, in some cases, suffer with their own specific problems. For example, CT scans are often insensitive to very subtle changes in brain structure, while MRI scans can over-estimate CNS involvement in certain conditions and can even produce artefacts known as unidentified bright objects (UBOs), which are of uncertain origin and, at present, thought to be the tangential cross-sectional images of gyri and sulci (the convolutions and grooves observed on the surface of the brain).

For the neuropsychologist, then, having an understanding of these principles and at least a working knowledge of the investigations used, ensures that the patient's evaluation is not solely dependent on the neuroimaging results.

PLAIN FILM RADIOGRAPHY (X-RAY)

Despite the advances in imaging processes over the last 30 years, the plain film radiograph still represents a useful tool in the preliminary investigation

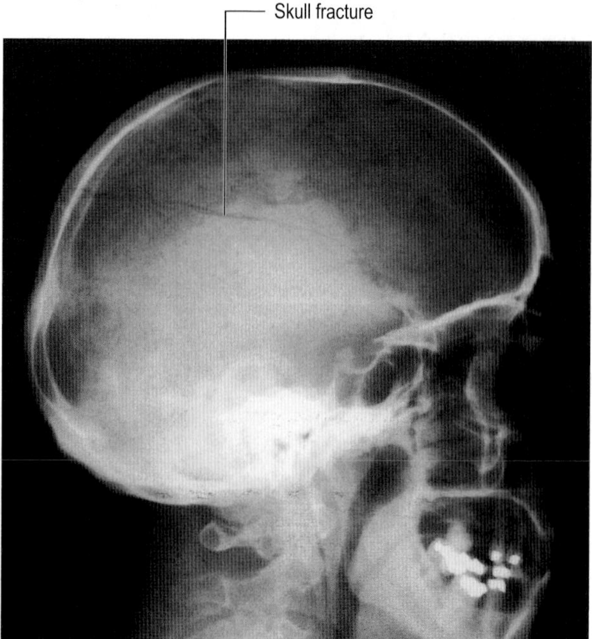

Fig. 4.1 X-ray of the head showing a fracture of the skull. (From Drake et al 2005, p 780)

of cases involving head trauma, bone erosion and the secondary effects of raised intracranial pressure. X-rays are high energy electromagnetic waves composed of particles known as photons. These photons are capable of penetrating the body but lose more energy as they pass through increasingly dense tissue. Thus, when captured on photographic film, low density areas, such as CSF, appear dark because they do not absorb a great deal of energy while high density areas, such as bone, appear light. Figure 4.1 demonstrates this pattern of light and dark or high and low attenuation and shows clearly the presence of a skull fracture.

In addition to fractures, then, such images, taken from a variety of different angles, can be used to look for bone erosion, abnormal calcification, and signs of raised intracranial pressure. Unfortunately, however, X-rays are a harmful form of ionizing radiation and there is a limit to the number of exposures a patient can safely have in a given time. Furthermore, the X-ray does not, given its relative insensitivity, rule out other forms of significant disease processes and more subtle trauma.

COMPUTED TOMOGRAPHY (CT)

Since the 1970s the development of non-invasive scanning techniques has revolutionized our approach to investigative pathology and it is now a routine form of procedure. In computed tomography (CT) scanning a focused beam of X-rays is rotated around the head while a fixed array of detectors is used to measure the degree of absorption by the tissues. Again the relative density of the tissues through which the X-rays pass determines the amount of energy lost by the individual X-ray photon and, thus, can be used as a foundation from which a computer can develop a two-dimensional image (Fig. 4.2).

In routine scanning the CT produces images at every 5 to 10 mm. For higher resolution scans, images can be produced at between 1 and 2 mm, although this is a somewhat more difficult and time-consuming process and is, therefore, usually reserved for specific investigations. To further enhance these images, for example when a plain scan is suggestive of the presence of an abnormality or if the patient's presentation is suggestive of the presence of a specific pathology such as an arteriovenous malformation, an intravenous or intrathecal contrast medium can be introduced. Still further CT scan images can now be used, with the addition of sophisticated computer software, to produce three-dimensional images which can be rotated on the computer screen to better visualize cerebral pathology.

Obviously the advantages of such advancements in radiography over the plain film radiograph are enormous in that CT scanning, for the first time, allowed us to visualize the softer tissues within the skull without the use of an invasive technique. Moreover, it allowed for the early detection of patholo-

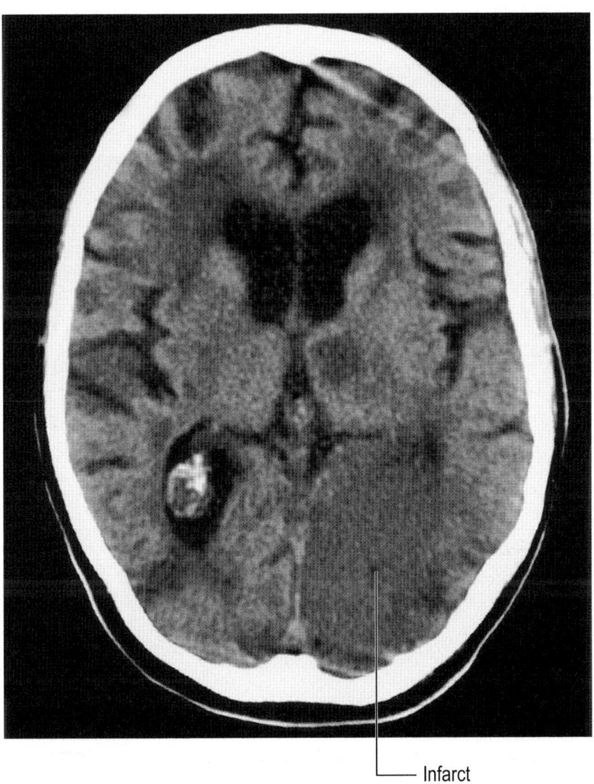

Fig. 4.2 CT scan of the brain showing a cerebral infarct. (From Drake et al 2005, p 791)

gies that, hitherto, would have gone undetected until much later in the course of the disease. Unfortunately, however, CT scanning is still based on the use of potentially harmful ionizing radiation which, therefore, limits the individual degree of the patient's exposure. It is also of a lower resolution than other scanning techniques and insensitive to certain types of pathology.

MAGNETIC RESONANCE IMAGING (MRI)

First referred to as nuclear magnetic resonance imaging (NMRI), the prefix 'nuclear' being abandoned early on because of the emotive link with radiation, magnetic resonance imaging (MRI) detects the motion of hydrogen protons within a magnetic field in response to electromagnetic pulses. Essentially, the patient lies within the scanner and a strong magnetic field ensures that the freely spinning protons align with the magnetic field, much like a compass needle responds to a magnet. Next, an electromagnetic pulse, a radiowave, is passed through the patient's head and the consequent reverberations in the aligned protons are detected by the scanner (Fig. 4.3).

T_1-weighted MRI scans detect the time taken for the reverberating protons to realign themselves with the magnetic field (using the compass analogy, the time taken for the compass needle to settle back to the magnet if the compass is shaken). T_2-weighted scans detect the time taken for the reverberating protons to return to their free rotating state (again using the example of a compass, the time taken for the needle to settle once the magnet is taken away).

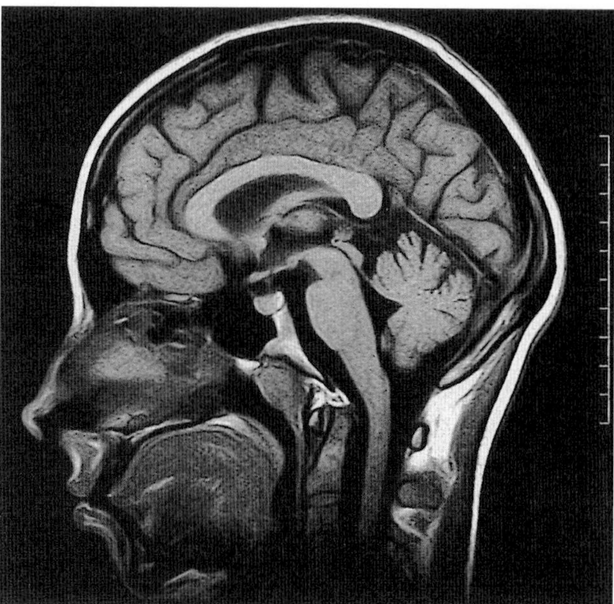

Fig. 4.3 T_1-weighted MRI scan of the brain. (Courtesy of Professor A. Jackson, Department of Diagnostic Radiology, University of Manchester. From Crossman & Neary 2000, p 31)

When looking at Figure 4.3, it is easy to see the advantages of MRI over CT scanning in that the process offers higher resolution images of the brain. However, MRI is also more adaptive than CT in that it can offer different sectional views of the brain in any plane, something that CT cannot. It is also more sensitive to changes in the soft tissues of the brain and, most importantly, offers no risk from repeated exposure to ionizing radiation.

In terms of the disadvantages of this investigation procedure, however, MRI, because of the use of strong magnetic fields, cannot be used with patients with pacemakers or other ferromagnetic implants. At around 3 mm, MRI is also limited in the thickness of image slices it can produce when compared to CT scanning and does not produce good visualization of bone. Furthermore, MRI scanning is prone to artefacts caused by movement of the patient during the procedure and can be difficult to employ if the patient to be scanned is claustrophobic as the scanner itself requires the individual to be enclosed in a somewhat noisy tubular chamber.

FUNCTIONAL MAGNETIC RESONANCE IMAGING (FMRI)

Utilizing the same technology as MRI, functional magnetic resonance imaging (fMRI) relies on changes in the magnetic properties of haemoglobin caused by oxygen concentration changes in the blood and thus, instead of producing structural images of the brain, provides important functional data with regard to functional changes in the tissues. In the early days of research in this area, paramagnetic enhancement substances such as gadolinium were used to augment MRI images, and even today can be used for the investigation of ischaemia, demyelination and tumours. However, the more recent and non-invasive blood oxygenation level dependent contrast technique has become the norm for functional assessment.

Briefly, local changes in the level of cellular activity within the brain result in a change in cerebral blood flow and the use of oxygen by the tissues. In turn, this has a direct effect on the levels of oxygenated and deoxygenated haemoglobin, which contain different forms of iron. The resultant changes in the local magnetic field can then be measured by the scanner and a pattern of function visualized. Thus, patterns of activation can be detected and images corresponding to a variety of cognitive, sensory or motor tasks produced.

SINGLE PHOTON EMISSION COMPUTED TOMOGRAPHY (SPECT)

Again looking at the functional aspects of the brain as opposed to its structure, single photon emission computed tomography (SPECT) relies on the introduction of a radioactive isotope emitting gamma photons and the subsequent detection of these gamma photons by an array of detectors. The isotope compound can be administered intravenously or orally, or can be inhaled in the form of a gas, and is chosen for its particular biochemical properties in that it will tend to bind to receptor sites in the brain, or be taken up by the bones, heart or kidneys. The most frequently used compound hexamethylpropyleneamine oxime (HMPAO) is used as the tracer in studies of cerebral blood flow. Once again computers are used to collect the data from the detectors and to produce a two-dimensional or three-dimensional image based on the level of receptor site activity and, in terms of brain imaging, provide information on cellular activity and perfusion.

Clinically, SPECT has been useful in the assessment of blood flow in cerebrovascular disease, dementia, and in the evaluation of patients with intractable epilepsy. Unfortunately, however, SPECT has a lower image resolution than both CT and MRI.

POSITRON EMISSION TOMOGRAPHY (PET)

The positron emission tomography (PET) technique relies upon the positron emission properties of a number of isotopes which are, in turn, bound to biologically useful compounds to make a quantitative study of the brain's use of metabolites such as oxygen or glucose, or changes in cerebral blood flow. Thus, each decaying positron gives off two photons travelling in opposite directions, which then set off a pair of diametrically opposed detectors. The output of such an array of detectors is then processed by a computer and an image similar to that of a CT is produced.

PET is particularly useful in the investigation of the relationship between blood flow and oxygen use in the brain, and therefore, has been used to study patients with focal ischaemia and infarct, as well as dementia, epilepsy and brain tumour. Unfortunately, however, because of the nature of the equipment used, PET can be relatively expensive to undertake, and again, relies on radiation to obtain imaging data, thus limiting individual exposure.

Finally, PET scans, because of the relatively short half-life of the isotopes used, often do not produce enough specific data for a single individual to provide a picture of brain activity. In practice, however, PET studies often involve an averaging across a number of individuals and so a great deal of the work undertaken with this type of imaging technology is in the field of research rather than clinical application.

ELECTROENCEPHALOGRAPHY (EEG)

Through the use of scalp electrodes, electroencephalography (EEG) assesses electrical activity in the brain. Small electrical potentials, measuring less than 100 microvolts, are recorded and amplified. Filters then remove unwanted high and low frequency signals, such as the electrical activity caused by muscular movement, and the results are displayed as a series of waves by either a pen recorder or on a computer monitor (Fig. 4.4). The EEG, then, records both the resting pattern of electrical brain activity as well as the reaction of the patient under conditions such as hyperventilation or during photic stimulation with a flashing stroboscopic light, which may result in the discharges of brain activity common in epilepsy. In telemetric recording a con-

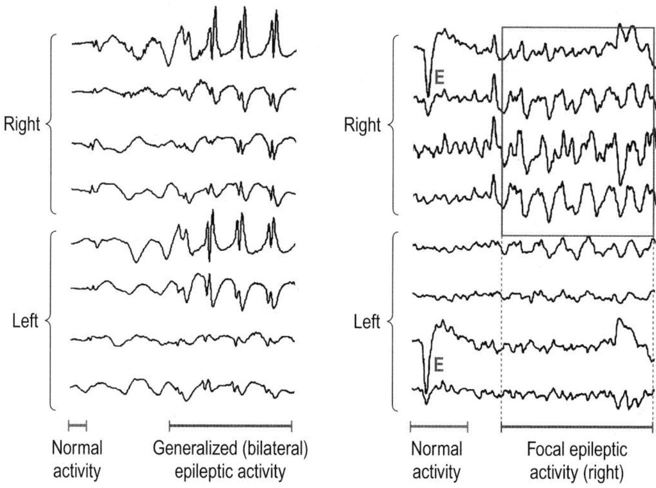

Fig. 4.4 EEG waves. (From Kumar & Clark 2005, p 1203)

tinuous 24 or 48 hour recording of brain activity is made and is often combined with video recording of the patient.

The EEG is divided into four main wavebands categorized by their frequency. These wavebands include beta (13–22 Hz), alpha (8–12 Hz), theta (5–7 Hz), and delta (1–4 Hz) and these vary with the patient's level of alertness and wakefulness. In a person who is awake and alert, frequencies in the beta waveband predominate. However, when a person is relaxed with eyes closed, slower frequencies in the alpha waveband are most common. By contrast, during sleep, very low frequencies in the delta waveband are observed (such characteristic EEG patterns, then, can be used to detect and diagnose problems such as sleep disorders).

In epilepsy, however, the normal synchronous firing of brain cells producing these wave frequencies is often disrupted by large, random discharges or 'spikes'. In turn, these are recorded as rapid changes in wave activity on the EEG recording. The effects of anticonvulsant medication for epilepsy can also be seen on the EEG as a reduction in this spiking activity.

Clinically, the EEG is non-invasive and relatively inexpensive. It can be used to measure brain activity in real time and has the advantage of being repeatable without harmful effects to the patient. Unfortunately, EEGs are also susceptible to artefacts caused by movement and may be poor in terms of specific functional localization.

ANGIOGRAPHY

Many neurological conditions require the accurate assessment of the blood vessels both inside and outside the brain. In angiography, an arterial injection of a contrast medium, given under local or general anaesthetic, is imaged

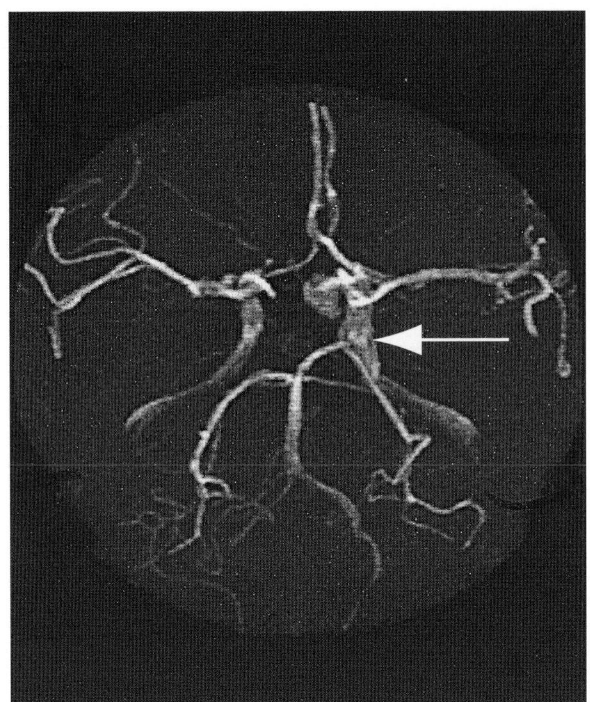

Fig. 4.5 DSA angiogram of posterior communicating artery aneurysm. (From Kumar & Clark 2005, p 1217)

with either a standard X-ray film or, in the case of digital subtraction angiography (DSA), an image processor and display unit.

In cerebral angiography, a catheter is inserted into the femoral artery and moved to the carotid or vertebral arteries. Contrast is then injected via a high pressure pump and a series of X-ray films exposed in order to visualize the travel of the contrast medium through the vessels. In the case of DSA, exposures both before and after the administration of the contrast medium are subtracted from one another by computer. The resulting image allows for the enhancement of smaller differences between images to be investigated as well as providing the ability to magnify specific areas. Overall, such improved contrast sensitivity permits the use of lower concentrations of contrast materials (Fig. 4.5).

SUMMARY

Prior to the advent of sophisticated scanning procedures, clinicians were limited to a handful of non-invasive investigations including EEG, X-ray and neuropsychological assessment. While these tests still have their place, the last 30 years has seen the development and establishment of more complex and precise procedures including: CT, MRI and DSA, as well as the growth of functional measures such as fMRI, SPECT and PET. Nevertheless, it should also be noted that, while all of these improvements in imaging represent a substantial step forward in the diagnosis and treatment of neurological disorders, they each still suffer with their own problems and disadvantages.

REFERENCES

Crossman A R, Neary D 2000 Neuroanatomy. Churchill Livingstone, Edinburgh, p 31

Drake R L, Vogl W, Mitchell A W M 2005 Gray's Anatomy for Students. Churchill Livingstone, Edinburgh, p 780, 791

Kumar P, Clark M 2005 Clinical medicine, 6th edn. Elsevier Saunders, Edinburgh, p 1203, 1217

FURTHER READING

Dougherty D D, Rauch S L, Rosenbaum J 2004 Essentials of neuroimaging for clinical practice. American Psychiatric Publishing, Washington DC

Cabeza R, Kingstone A (eds) 2001 Handbook of functional neuroimaging of cognition. MIT Press, Cambridge

Emotional and psychological reactions

5

OVERVIEW

Before we go on to study in detail the more common disorders encountered by neuropsychologists, it might be useful to outline some of the general psychological and emotional effects that these disorders can produce. This will serve to provide both a background to each condition and a context within which to assess pathological responses. In this section, then, we will look at the more typical individual processes involved and also briefly examine the wider scope of the reactions of family and/or carers.

PSYCHOLOGICAL AND EMOTIONAL REACTIONS

The onset of any traumatic event has a sudden, unexpected, and tremendously pervasive effect on the individual's life, creating psychological and emotional imbalance. However, in the case of injuries or illness involving the central nervous system, this effect is, perhaps, amplified because it strikes at the very core of what defines our lives – our memories, personalities, and so on.

Unlike many debilitating diseases, such as arthritis, brain damage, more often than not, happens very suddenly and offers the sufferer no chance for gradual adaptation to the condition. The patient, therefore, and the family and carers are commonly forced into a situation where they must quickly adjust not only to the stress of acute and possibly life-threatening illness but also to the often confusing physical and psychological disabilities that accompany the condition.

Depression and anxiety

Broadly speaking, the most immediate and common reactions to such a trauma are, not surprisingly, depression, anxiety and grief. It should be noted, however, that these emotions are not only experienced simply within the isolation of the acute phase of a shock reaction but permeate almost every facet of the everyday life of patients and their carers.

This is because, with the passage of time, it often becomes clear that there may have to be radical alterations in life-style, social and economic status, employment and even the capacity to maintain relationships. For the sufferer and the carer alike, social activities may become difficult if not impossible to pursue. Work or business endeavours might be cut short. Hobbies and interests may have to be abandoned.

Emotional reactions to these circumstances, then, are fairly easy to understand. For the patient there might be feelings of uselessness, loss of self-esteem, frustration and so on. For the family or carers there may be feelings of guilt, frustration, isolation, or similar expressions of anxiety or depression.

In the individual, such feelings commonly conspire to produce an introspective, uncommunicative and withdrawn state, where the patient may be unwilling or unable to cooperate because of feelings of sheer hopelessness. Or, if a strong element of frustration is associated with the depression or anxiety, there may be episodes of resentment and anger that punctuate the presentation.

On an individual basis, however, it must be remembered that these displays of emotion are, in themselves, to be expected. In fact, they can even be viewed as quite encouraging since, despite the obvious distress involved, such emotional reactions tend to indicate that the essential function of comprehension is largely unimpaired. Conversely, where these reactions do not occur, it is possible that the patient is unaware or does not understand what is happening to them.

Grief

Grief, on the other hand, is a natural reaction to a loss of any kind. For example, grief may be felt for the death of a loved one or the loss of a relationship. However, it should also be remembered that one may even experience grief for the loss of an ability or even the loss of a potential; that is to say the loss of something that has not yet been achieved.

Essentially a process of adaptation, grief passes through a number of fairly well-defined stages that are displayed to different degrees in different people. These stages include: alarm, shock, denial, mitigation, anger, guilt, acceptance and adjustment. These stages of reaction are a normal and essential part of the process of adaptation. To some extent they are protective and defensive and provide the patient with time for mental healing. So the carer should generally go along with them up to a point, remembering that the patient should not become trapped at any one stage, thus allowing the development of a long-term pathological emotional response.

In practice, not all of these stages will be immediately recognizable and very often they overlap. It is important, therefore, not to think of this model as a fixed, individual response pattern, but as a general guide to what may be expected. It is also important to remember that different people may progress through these various stages at different rates. Progress from one stage to the next cannot be considered to be smooth and continuous.

In the presence of a neurological disorder, however, grief reactions are very much more complex than those experienced during, say, bereavement. This is because the loss in this context may be very much more abstract than the loss of a specific object such as a person. Whereas in bereavement, the cycle of grieving can largely be completed, the loss incurred with physical or neuropsychological disability remains an integral part of everyday life. While the bereaved person may come to terms with the loss and eventually close the gap left by the death of a loved one, the person grieving for the loss of, for instance the ability to communicate intelligibly, must learn to live with the gap left by the dysfunction every day.

Role loss and role change

For the individual patient, grief, depression and anxiety will be experienced as a reaction to a multitude of factors, including loss of role, changes in role and changes in the self-concept.

Roles are socially defined behavioural expectations for individuals occupying certain social positions and for those who interact with them. Most transitions in life are accompanied by role changes, and these changes involve either gains, for example being promoted or getting married, or losses, for example getting divorced or retiring. Role change can, therefore, be more or less difficult depending on whether the new role involves either a loss or a gain, or whether the new role is perceived as positive or negative. To illustrate, we have used the example of retirement, above, to describe a negative role change. However, many of us view retirement as a positive role change.

In the case of an individual suffering, for example, a stroke, we can see that the various roles played by the person before and after the event may vary greatly. For instance, before the stroke the patient may have been: husband/wife, father/mother, employee, social club member and driver. All these roles possess many positive aspects. After the event, however, because of the disabling effects of brain injury, we see that the patient's rich diversity of roles has been reduced to: husband/wife, father/mother and stroke victim.

So the effect for this patient, not surprisingly, is not only a drastic reduction in the variety and richness of premorbid roles but also the addition or transition to a new role, that of stroke victim: a role that may symbolize a great many negative life factors.

Apart from these very obvious problems, role loss and role change can also produce a variety of other difficulties through conflicts and confusion in the expectations of others. For example, patients who are hospitalized may be expected to assume the sick role, even if they themselves wish to maintain as much control over their lives as possible. Conversely, the reverse may also occur when patients may be expected to resume premorbid roles while they, in fact, are still adjusting to the role of patient and still needing comfort and support.

The roles associated with the personal and societal expectations of one's chronological age can also provide a source of stress in the adjustment process. For example, an individual of 20 years who is living at home with their parents will experience a great deal less social stress than an individual of 45 years in the same situation. This is because age carries with it social expectations for development.

Thus, patients who are constrained in their normal adult development at a given age must come to terms with not only a deviation from the societal norm but also the loss of potential future developments and role transitions.

In early adulthood, then, we observe task and experience gains associated with that stage of role development. Typically, there is the forming of new relationships, the development of self-reliance, the forging of a career path, the setting of long-term life goals, a separation from parents, an increased mobility and financial independence. Frustration of the individual's ability to fulfil these role tasks and experience gains can, therefore, cause profound psychological and emotional disturbance.

As the normal progression through these developmental stages continues, the tasks and experience vary, but the potentialities of arrested development remain the same. Here we see some of the tasks and experiences of someone in later life, which might include an adjustment to retirement, adjustment to a reduced income, a re-interpretation of life goals and aims, a consolidation of relationships, adjustment to the death of parents, coping with reduced mobility and adjustment to the physiological changes associated with ageing.

Importantly, however, while the focus of emotional disturbance will be different for the age groupings used in these examples, the resultant emotional impact caused by cerebral dysfunction and consequent disability will be essentially the same.

Changes in the self-concept

The self-concept is a subjective mental picture of who we are. It consists of a collection of beliefs about what we think we are like. The self-concept might include such beliefs as: I am fat, I am shy, or I am friendly. A good exercise to try is compiling a list of one's own beliefs about oneself. It should be possible to see from the resultant list of self-referent beliefs that the self-concept includes many aspects, amongst which are our physical, social, emotional and intellectual selves.

Derived from these various aspects of our own make-up, we each crucially possess a dimension of self-evaluation that is, all the time, re-evaluating the way we appear to ourselves and others. Another good exercise to undertake is to try to evaluate the social element of these self-evaluations by making the same list of self-referent beliefs with a group of friends. Generally, we tend to moderate our responses and play down the positive when faced with a social group.

As a consequence of our self-evaluations we generally appraise ourselves in either an approving or disapproving manner. As a result of these favourable or unfavourable self-evaluations our level of self-esteem is determined. Self-esteem, the global self-evaluation of one's worth as a person, is probably the most important element of the self-concept, and the importance of a positive attitude towards oneself cannot be overestimated.

For neurologically impaired patients the loss or reduction of self-esteem can be an extremely important factor in their emotional response to all facets of treatment, rehabilitation, family life, social interaction, and so on. Therefore, when encountering patients whose intellect may be dulled, who might have difficulty in communicating, who display memory problems, or who have poor mobility, it is not surprising to learn that they will be prone to negative self-evaluation in terms of their own self-image perceptions, the way in which they feel others perceive them, and indeed in their perception of the person they would like to be.

In practice, this usually means that patients will become depressed, anxious, self-conscious, and introverted. They may lose self-confidence, lack motivation, withdraw socially and ultimately set low goals for achievement because they assume that they cannot succeed, even with effort. Ultimately, their ability to cope with their circumstances is reduced and their sense of helplessness becomes a self-fulfilling prophecy.

COPING PROCESSES

In addition to these various emotional changes are a number of coping processes and cognitive adjustments that patients may exhibit as they gradually adjust to their disabilities.

Patients, then, will often display either an emotion-focused form of coping, a problem-focused form of coping, or a mixture of both. Emotion-focused coping involves the use of emotions to deal with the trauma and the regulation of emotional responses, and can, for example, be observed as denial, distraction, or the seeking of social support. Problem-focused coping, on the other hand, involves action to alter the problem, such as seeking further information regarding a particular condition.

There are a number of specific cognitive processes that patients may use to cope with trauma. Some of the most common of these are to find meaning in an event, to gain control over a situation or condition, and to restore self-esteem.

To illustrate, patients suffering from a stroke may try to find meaning in their experiences by attributing causation, either by determining why their stroke came about or by rethinking their attitudes and priorities.

Depending on the individual reaction, the effect of this can be either positive or negative. For example, patients may attribute causation to their premorbid smoking habit and thus gain a better understanding of the pathogenesis of their condition. They may even change their future behaviour in the light of this knowledge and prevent such a behaviour from contributing to future health problems. Conversely, other patients may view their condition as a form of punishment for previous deeds or thoughts, a particularly difficult obstacle to overcome in treatment and rehabilitation.

Many patients also attempt to gain a sense of control over their condition. They may try to increase their level of knowledge, thus making themselves more aware and subjectively more in control. Or they may throw themselves wholeheartedly into the rehabilitation process and gain another measure of control. In contrast, Seligman (1974) described a syndrome termed 'learned helplessness'. This model of depression involves passivity produced by prolonged exposure to unavoidable events. Thus, in situations where control is not perceived by the patient, as is often the case with neurological trauma, it is not unusual to observe a withdrawal or a reduction in motivation.

Finally, patients may attempt to restore a certain level of self-esteem by comparing themselves to others, usually those less fortunate, or with comparator scenarios. For example, patients may compare themselves to other individuals with more widespread neurological damage, or might describe their own situation as being worse if some factor was not present.

Family and carer processes

It is imperative to bear in mind that the vast majority of the individual patients that we work with are also members of families or groups who, generally speaking, will become the providers of long-term care and support. Inevitably, then, the patient will have an effect on this unit as will other members of the unit on the patient.

In order to adapt to a member with a disability, families as units, generally speaking, appear to have to work through the same or similar stages of grieving as the patient. Very briefly, these stages include:

- *Shock*: family members often report feelings of confusion, numbness, disorganization and helplessness. Often they feel that they were unable to take in much of the information they were given regarding the diagnosis, etc.
- *Denial*: disbelief of the reality of the situation. As was the case for the patient, this stage offers the family a temporary defence against the initial shock.
- *Anger*: family members will often seek a cause for the condition of the patient and may end up blaming themselves or a multitude of other factors for the situation. More often than not this anger will become displaced onto other family members, causing further tension. It may even be directed to the professionals involved in the case.
- *Sadness*: as with the individual, family members may exhibit depression or despair.
- *Detachment*: at this point, family members often experience a time when they feel empty. Nothing seems to matter. They are resigned to the reality of the situation but appear to have lost some of the energy and involvement observed in the earlier stages.
- *Re-organization*: this stage is usually characterized by realism and the development of hope for the patient's future.
- *Adaptation*: finally, when family members have come to terms with the situation, they will often exhibit an emotional acceptance of the disabled family member. They are aware of the patient's special needs and try to provide for them.

As can be seen, there are great similarities to the individual's process of adjustment, at least as far as the staging of the process is concerned. However, it is important within this apparent parallel process to distinguish between the focus of the grief reaction for family members and for the patient.

First, it is obvious that each individual will probably exhibit a different emphasis on different aspects of the situation at different times. Thus, if the family members and the individual patient are at different stages of the grieving and adaptation process, they might be of little assistance to each other. For instance, if family members are still in a state of denial while the individual is struggling with anger over their loss, there can be a tremendous impact on family life, leaving little room for constructive communication.

Secondly, the losses for different family members, though based on the same event, will not be the same. For instance, the parents of a young adult suffering a stroke might mourn the loss of their newly acquired freedom from the full-time parenting role. The siblings of the same patient, however, might, at the same time, be experiencing anger at having to assume a caretaker role.

COMMON FAMILY AND CARER PROBLEMS

Despite their own emotional difficulties, the family will still play an important role in achieving adjustment for the patient. However, this can only be of benefit if the family members themselves are able to adjust. Below is a list of just a few of the most common problems experienced by the families of severely brain-damaged individuals:

- A lack of information concerning possible outcomes
- Mourning and accepting the loss of the patient's premorbid personality
- Adjusting to the patient's lack of insight
- Feelings of guilt over the cause or inability to prevent the accident/illness
- Dealing with the emotional consequences of the trauma or illness
- Adjustment to the responsibility of long-term care of the patient
- Time and attention investment needed for rehabilitation
- Acceptance of an uncertain future
- Adjusting to a reduced level of income
- A loss of social contacts.

Naturally, the emotional consequences of such stresses and strains, in concert with the upheaval of the early stages of the adaptation process, can often produce a breakdown in family relationships. It is needless to say, therefore, that these tensions serve only to reduce the likelihood of positive outcomes.

SUMMARY

The emotional and psychological consequences of neurological illness and trauma cannot be over-stated. Such imbalances in normal psychoemotional functioning are the inevitable result of illness or trauma that strike at the very fabric of what each of us cherishes as unique and individual.

For the patient and the family alike, it is to be expected that a degree of anxiety and depression will be experienced before acceptance and adjustment can be achieved in the grieving process. As the process of adaptation progresses, there may be complications due to the multifaceted psychosocial and psychophysiological aspects of the losses incurred.

Loss and circumscription of roles and changes in the self-concept may lead to negative self-evaluations and a reduction in the self-esteem in the individual. The family and carers of the victim, on the other hand, may also suffer their own parallel emotional and psychological difficulties as well as practical difficulties which, while distressing in their own right, may also have a further impact on the patient.

REFERENCE

Seligman M E P 1974 Depression and learned helplessness. In: Friedman R J, Katz M (eds) The psychology of depression. Contemporary theory and research. Wiley, New York

FURTHER READING

Fraser R T, Clemmons D C 1999 Traumatic brain injury rehabilitation: practical vocational, neuropsychological, and psychotherapy interventions. CRC Press, Boca Raton

Langer K G, Lewis L, Laatsch L 1999 Psychotherapeutic interventions for adults with brain injury or stroke: a clinician's treatment resource. Psychosocial Press, Madison

Wood R L, Wood T 2000 Neurobehavioural disability and social handicap following traumatic brain injury. Psychology Press, Philadelphia

The neuropsychology of common disorders

6

OVERVIEW

The preceding chapters will have provided a basic grounding in neuropsychology, functional neuroanatomy and some of the more common neuroimaging techniques, as well as introducing some of the psychological and emotional processes that might be observed in neurological populations.

The following chapter is divided into separate sections dealing with specific disorders and seeks to build on the different factors highlighted within the preceding material to present a brief introduction to some of the more commonly encountered neuropsychological presentations associated with these. To this end we will examine more closely Alzheimer's disease and some of the other dementing conditions, cerebral vascular accident (CVA) or stroke, epilepsy, multiple sclerosis, Parkinson's disease, parkinsonism and the Parkinson's plus syndromes, and traumatic brain injury.

Each subsection contains a short overview and description of the disorder, pathology, aetiology and epidemiology. It will offer a review of the more frequent neuropsychological symptoms observed in these cases and a summary.

ALZHEIMER'S DISEASE AND THE OTHER DEMENTIAS

Overview

Alzheimer's disease, although the most frequently encountered dementing process, is only one of a number of conditions causing a progressive and widespread decline in neuropsychological functioning. Here, then, while we will look primarily at Alzheimer's disease, we will also attempt to summarize some of the presenting factors of the other major disorders, such as multi-infarct or vascular dementia.

Description

Dementia is a debilitating syndrome. It is a collection of symptoms that may or may not point to a disease, but is not a disease entity in itself (Selby 2000). The term is used to refer to a global deterioration of higher mental functioning in clear consciousness that is beyond that which might be expected to occur in normal ageing. It is progressive and usually irreversible.

Although an individual can become demented following acute neurological trauma, dementia is typically a progressive condition, developing through stages. Usually these stages are characterized as mild, moderate or severe. In the mild stage, patients generally retain judgement and may be able to maintain their independence. In the moderate stage, independence cannot be maintained and some degree of supervision is required. As the condition progresses to the severe stage, patients will become extremely impaired and require constant supervision. Finally, and sadly inevitably, the condition will lead to death.

The most obvious neuropsychological manifestations include: disruption of memory (long-term and short-term), disruption of language processes (nominal aphasia being most common) disruption of intellectual skills, personality change, behavioural change, apathy and/or depression, psychotic phenomena (delusions of persecution, hallucination).

However, while the dementias all lead to the same point, they present differently in terms of behavioural and cognitive symptom presentation, and their course. Broadly, therefore, the dementias can be divided into four categories: cortical dementias (e.g. Alzheimer's disease, frontal lobe disease, Creutzfeldt-Jakob disease), subcortical dementias (e.g. Huntington's disease, Parkinson's disease), mixed variety dementias (e.g. multi-infarct dementia, acquired immunodeficiency syndrome (AIDS)-related complex), and reversible dementias.

The cortical dementias represent the most well-known group of disorders as they tend to affect those more obvious cognitive abilities associated with the cortex. The subcortical dementias, however, are somewhat more obscure in that these generally affect areas of the brain which, at least in the earlier stages, do not result in the more conspicuous cognitive deficits. Mixed-variety dementias are conditions which, as is clear from the title given to this group, appear to have both a cortical and a subcortical component. Finally, the reversible dementias are represented by a host of conditions that can cause dementia or dementia-like symptoms. As the name implies, this group consists of conditions which, by and large, mimic dementia but that are generally amenable to treatment. These include infections, reactions to medications, metabolic and endocrine disorders, cardiac and respiratory disorders, nutritional deficiencies, exposure to toxins, the use and abuse of recreational intoxicants such as alcohol, and depression.

Obviously, an exhaustive examination of all these dementing conditions, their epidemiology, aetiology, and neurobehavioural presentation is not possible here. With the exception of depression and reversible dementia, which will be examined in more detail in Chapter 7, what follows is a brief summary with regard to the most common forms of dementia encountered.

Epidemiology

According to the Alzheimer's Society, dementia, as a whole, affects approximately 750 000 people in the UK, with over 18 000 of these individuals being aged less than 65 years. Statistically, dementia affects around 1 person in 20 aged over 65 years and one person in 5 over 80 years of age. As a result of increasing life expectancy, it has been estimated that the total number of sufferers in the UK will rise to around 870 000 by the year 2010 and some 1.8 million by the year 2050.

By far the most common is Alzheimer's disease (AD), which was named after Dr Alois Alzheimer, the first to observe the tell-tale abnormal amyloid plaques and neurofibrillary tangles in the brain. There are some 600 000 sufferers in the UK. More prevalent than CVA for healthy individuals aged between 75 years and 85 years in the Western hemisphere (Lovenstone & Ritchie 2002), AD accounts for some 55% of dementias and is the fourth most common cause of death, equally as prevalent as myocardial infarction.

In general the symptoms of AD appear after the age of 60 years. There are, however, some early-onset forms of the disease and these are usually linked to a specific gene defect. AD causes a gradual decline in cognitive abilities and the average life expectancy of patients subsequent to diagnosis is 7 to 10 years (although some patients have been known to live up to 20 years from their diagnosis).

Vascular dementia or multi-infarct dementia (MID) is the second most common cause of dementia after AD and accounts for around 20% of all dementias. It is caused by damage resulting from cerebrovascular or cardiovascular problems and is often associated with CVA. In many cases, vascular dementia may coexist with AD and its incidence increases with advancing age. The ratio of occurrence between males and females is roughly similar.

The symptoms of vascular dementia are often acute in onset, frequently occurring after a CVA. Indeed, patients may demonstrate many of the same risk factors as in a CVA. The associated dementia may or may not progress depending on the occurrence of additional CVAs. When the condition does progress, as might be expected, the mechanism of progressive damage often produces a stepwise decline, associated with sudden changes, rather than the steady degeneration observed in other dementias.

There are several types of vascular dementia, which vary in their aetiology and symptom presentation. These include Binswanger's disease (also known as subcortical arteriosclerotic leukoencephalopathy) and cerebral autosomal dominant arteriopathy with subcortical infarct and leukoencephalopathy (CADASIL), a rare genetic disorder.

Lewy body dementia (LBD) shares some of the characteristics of AD but can also be observed in some cases of Parkinson's disease (PD). Affecting both men and women equally, the condition, as might be expected, is more prevalent in those over the age of 65 years and probably accounts for around 15% of all dementia cases. It is, therefore, one of the most common forms of progressive dementia.

LBD generally occurs sporadically, with the development of Lewy bodies in the cells of the substantia nigra (see the later section on PD). These abnormal structures may also appear in the cortex and contain a protein called alpha-synuclein that has been linked to PD and several other disorders, prompting some to refer to these disorders collectively as synucleinopathies.

On average, patients with a diagnosis of LBD survive for some 7 years after symptoms present.

Frontal lobe disease or frontotemporal dementia (FTD) is an umbrella term for a number of conditions that appear to be restricted to the frontotemporal areas of the brain. This includes Pick's disease, frontal lobe degeneration and the dementia associated with motor neuron disease. FTD is rare, accounting for approximately 5% of dementia cases, and while there appears to be no difference in the sex ratio of this condition, it does appear more likely to occur in those under the age of 65 years.

The symptoms of FTD usually appear between the ages of 40 years and 65 years. In many cases, patients with FTD demonstrate a family history of dementia, suggesting a genetic link. The course and duration of FTD varies widely. Some patients will decline rapidly over 2 to 3 years while some patients will show only minimal changes over the course of years. The life expectancy of patients with a new diagnosis of FTD is approximately 5 to 10 years.

Huntington's disease (HD) represents an hereditary, autosomal dominant disorder caused by a defective gene. The disease causes progressive degeneration in many regions of the brain and spinal cord. Symptoms of HD usually begin when patients are in their 30s or 40s, and the average life expectancy after diagnosis is about 15 years. The offspring of sufferers have a 50% chance of inheriting the disorder.

Creutzfeldt-Jakob disease (CJD), on the other hand, was until recently not a widely known cause of dementia. However, the weight of current media coverage has caused the condition, first defined in the 1920s, to become a matter of public interest. This is most probably because a new form of the disease, variant CJD (vCJD), was reported in 1996 which was linked to bovine spongiform encephalopathy (BSE) in cattle and the consumption of beef products.

CJD, however, is rare, affecting about one person per million every year. It can arise at any age but is most prevalent in those aged between 50 years and 60 years. Most cases of CJD occur sporadically, that is to say it occurs in individuals with no known risk factors for the disease. However, approximately 15% of cases demonstrate an hereditary factor. In very rare cases, CJD can also be acquired through exposure to diseased brain or nervous system tissue, usually through contamination via medical procedure. Life expectancy after diagnosis is approximately 1 year.

As regards vCJD, efforts have been made since 1989 to remove the causative protein contaminants from the human food chain and, indeed, there is now some evidence to suggest that the number of deaths from vCJD has reached a peak and that it is now in decline. Unfortunately, however, there is currently no definite means of predicting potential occurrences of vCJD and the future, therefore, remains uncertain. There could, for instance, be further cases that come to light over time as the incubation period for the causative protein agents remains uncertain and there may be a number of years from exposure to the development of symptoms.

The AIDS dementia complex (ADC) results from infection with the human immunodeficiency virus (HIV). HIV attacks the body's immune system, making the patient more susceptible to infection. AIDS-related cognitive impairment can occur, therefore, either as a direct impact of HIV on the brain or as the result of opportunist infections that take advantage of the weakened immune system. HIV, therefore, can both directly cause widespread damage to the white matter of the brain and compromise inmmunocompetence, resulting in parasitic, fungal and viral infections, tumour, and cerebrovascular damage.

It has been proposed that as many as 75 to 90% of patients dying from AIDS demonstrate cerebral pathology and that between 6 and 30% of patients will demonstrate dementia during the later stages of the illness (Banich 1997).

Finally, as we will see later, dementia may also occur in patients who have other disorders. The relationship between these disorders, however, and the presenting dementias is not always clear. Advanced PD is one such example. This can sometimes develop with symptoms of dementia and many Parkinson's patients may also have the amyloid plaques and neurofibrillary tangles found in AD. As yet, it is not known whether these two conditions may be linked or whether they simply co-exist in some patients.

Pathology

AD is characterized by two particular abnormalities: the presence of amyloid plaques and neurofibrillary tangles. These amyloid plaques and neurofibrillary tangles result in the death of nerve tissues in the brain and large numbers of these structures are considered diagnostic markers for AD.

Amyloid plaques are abnormal clusters of a protein that are found in the tissues outside neurons. The cores of amyloid plaques contain several proteins, the main one being known as amyloid β-peptide (Aβ), which is formed from a larger molecule, amyloid precursor protein (APP). Thus, abnormal APP metabolism can lead to excessive production of Aβ. This, although the underlying mechanism is not yet fully understood, is thought to represent a fundamental event that triggers AD.

Neurofibrillary tangles are bundles of twisted filaments found inside neurons. They form pairs of twisted filaments called paired helical filaments (PHF). PHFs are composed of a normal protein found in all neurons called tau. In normal cells, tau aids the functioning of structures known as microtubules, a part of the cell's structural support and transport network.

In AD, however, tau is changed such that it causes the formation of PHF tangles. When this happens, the microtubules cannot function correctly and they disintegrate. This collapse of the neuron's transport system may then impair communication between cells and cause them to die.

At present it is not known if these amyloid plaques and neurofibrillary tangles are primary or secondary. That is to say that, whether they themselves are harmful or if they occur as by-products of the disease process. What is known, however, is that as AD progresses, so the number of plaques and tangles observed increases.

In MID, impairment arises from ischaemia, haemorrhage or a cerebral insult resulting from cardiac arrest. Dementia results from the accumulation of numerous small cortical and subcortical infarcts and many of the risk factors for this condition are shared with CVA. The reader is, therefore, directed to the section on pathology under that heading. However, although not all CVAs cause dementia, it is the case that a single CVA can cause enough damage to the brain to cause dementia. This is known as single-infarct dementia.

By contrast, LBD presents with the same plaques and tangles as those observed in cases of AD. However, these cases also demonstrate the presence of abnormal structures known as Lewy bodies, structures containing a protein called alpha-synuclein.

Lewy bodies are found as coincidental pathology in a wide range of conditions including Down's syndrome, progressive supranuclear palsy and motor neuron disease, but are typically associated with idiopathic PD. The association of LBD with PD and AD has led to some confusion. The condition has been seen as a variant of both AD (Hansen et al 1990) and PD. However, it has also more recently been argued that LBD represents a clinically distinct entity.

Neuropathologically, FTD demonstrates an atrophy of the frontal and temporal lobes but the histological markers for AD, plaques and tangles, are absent. In Pick's disease, another form of less common dementia affecting the frontal lobes, a diagnostic histological marker is the presence of Pick bodies, which are degraded protein inclusions, named after their discoverer, and found within abnormal neural cells.

With HD, sufferers generally demonstrate a reduction in brain size of approximately 20% at post mortem. This cell loss is observed both cortically (Strange 1992) and subcortically, mainly in the caudate nucleus, and in the cerebellum. Positron emission tomography (PET) (Berent et al 1988) and computed tomography (CT) studies (Starkstein et al 1988) have shown both reduced metabolism and atrophy in the caudate nucleus. Accompanying this degeneration in HD is a concomitant derangement of the levels of many neurotransmitters.

Like HD, PD is considered to be a subcortical dementia. However, the neuropathology of PD is covered in some detail later in this chapter and, therefore, the reader is directed to that specific section of the text.

CJD, on the other hand, produces neuronal loss and vacuoles in the cytoplasm of neurons with a proliferation of glial cells. Histologically, there is a characteristic sponge-like appearance and the disorder, therefore, is known as a spongiform encephalopathy. In a small minority of cases, plaques resembling those in AD can be observed. These, however, do not appear to be composed of amyloid protein but prions (Kitamoto et al 1986). Conversely, in vCJD, these plaques and the expected spongiform changes appear to be widespread throughout the cortex (Will et al 1996).

Finally, as mentioned previously, ADC is rare and although a greater percentage of HIV sufferers demonstrate the virus in the central nervous system (CNS) at post mortem, the number of associated dementia cases is small. The mechanism of viral transport to the CNS is, as yet, unclear. However, once in the brain, the virus appears to cause the degeneration of neural tissue and particularly oligodendrocytes resulting in a loss of white matter (Navia et al 1986).

Aetiology

With regard to risk for the development of AD, increasing age is still seen as the most important factor. A family history of dementia is also known to increase risk (Terry & Katzman 1983). Other potential risk factors affecting the likelihood of developing AD that might interact with this genetic profile have also been put forward. These include female gender, exposure to the herpes simplex virus and a history of head trauma.

AD has also been linked to Down's syndrome. Chromosome 21 has been implicated in both AD and Down's syndrome (Jarvik 1988) and almost all patients with Down's syndrome who survive long enough demonstrate the signs of AD (Heston et al 1981). Moreover, it has been noted that Down's syndrome occurs more frequently in families with a history of AD and it has, therefore, been suggested that AD may be associated with the increasing age of the mother (Rocca et al 1986).

Exposure to toxic substances, such as organic solvents, or high levels of metals, such as aluminium, have also been proposed as a risk factor for the development of AD. However, the results of this aspect of the research have not been conclusive. For example, some evidence suggests heavy use of cigarettes could be a risk factor (Shalat et al 1987), while other studies claim that smoking may delay the presentation of symptoms.

Amongst the other factors claimed to relate to the incidence of AD have been viral transmission, alcoholism, the use of analgesics, levels of physical activity, and, believe it or not, nose picking (Herbert et al 1992). Even levels of education and the diversity and intensity of the range of activities undertaken in midlife have come under scrutiny.

It is very difficult, therefore, beyond the confirmed risks of age and genetics, to interpret the relative contribution of these associated factors. This suggests a multifactorial model in which individual factors interact with the environmental variables in determining the relative risk for the development of AD.

The list of factors involved in the development of MID is long and is, again, shared with many of the aetiological variables of CVA. Many cases of MID result from arteriosclerosis. However, other causes include cranial arteritis, systemic lupus erythematosus, sickle cell disease, hypertensive encephalopathy, menigovascular syphilis and tuberculous meningitis.

In LBD there is widespread cortical atrophy. This neuronal loss is observed throughout the cortex and especially in the temporal lobes. Subcortically there is also degeneration of the substantia nigra. Many of the remaining cortical and subcortical cells contain, as already mentioned, the Lewy bodies that are the hallmark of the disease. However, the mechanism by which these alpha-synuclein protein containing Lewy bodies accumulate is still unknown.

FTD produces a circumscribed cortical atrophy in the frontal and temporal lobes with neuronal loss, spongiform changes and gliosis but none of the plaques and tangles associated with AD. Cases of FTD are both familial and sporadic, which is to say that the degeneration occurs both as an hereditary disorder and spontaneously. The cause of sporadic FTD is still unknown.

HD is an autosomal dominant hereditary disorder and the offspring of a parent with HD have a 50% chance of inheriting the condition. The disease causes degeneration in many regions of the brain and spinal cord and is caused by a faulty gene on chromosome 4 which codes for a protein called huntingtin.

CJD occurs in three different ways: inherited, sporadic and iatrogenic. Inherited cases are secondary to mutations of the genes on chromosome 20 (Owen et al 1989) which control normal prion proteins. However, the mechanism involved in sporadic cases is not understood at present. It has been argued that these cases represent spontaneous age-related changes of the prion proteins into pathogenic forms, whereas others believe that these sporadic cases may, in fact, be infections with a very long incubation period (Galvez et al 1980). Iatrogenic cases of the disorder occur as a result of exposure to the tissues of CJD sufferers or equipment used in invasive CNS procedures with CJD patients. Causes for iatrogenic cases, therefore, can include such procedures as corneal transplants or injections of human growth hormone.

vCJD is a prion disorder acquired through the eating of infected beef products from livestock suffering from BSE (Moore 2001). However, there appears to be evidence that suggests host factors may be an important determinant for the development of the disease, in that all patients who have developed vCJD have possessed a normal genetic variant on the gene responsible for normal cellular prion proteins (Will et al 2000).

Overall, prions are extremely hardy and highly resistant to boiling, alcohol, formalin and even ultraviolet radiation. For example, electrodes used in a neurosurgical case with a patient suffering from CJD were still able to transmit the disorder to a chimpanzee some 2 years after their use, despite the fact that these items had been cleaned and were repeatedly sterilized with ethanol and formaldehyde vapour during the intervening period (Gibbs et al 1994).

As previously stated, ADC can occur after infection with HIV. The virus itself can be found in blood, semen, vaginal fluid and breast milk, and may be spread by contact with these fluids. Although the virus can be found in saliva, tears and urine, there is as yet no convincing evidence for transmission via these fluids. Sexual contact remains the predominant form of transmission for the virus. Blood-borne transmission remains a problem in intravenous drug use populations where there is a failure to sterilize needles but it is now rare in terms of the transfusion of blood, owing to improved screening techniques.

When HIV enters the body, the viral RNA is converted to DNA and inserted into the chromosomes of the host cells. When host cells divide, this DNA is copied and further viral RNA duplicates are made, which then leave the cell to infect other cells. The immune response initially contains this outbreak but does not eliminate the virus, which then continues to reproduce in the body's lymphoid tissue. The cell most likely to be infected is the T4 lymphocyte with the result that, over the course of years, the immune system becomes undermined and both the virus and other opportunistic infections take hold.

In ADC, then, the virus causes neuronal loss in the subcortical white matter and thalamus as well as atrophy in the cortex. Patients with a diagnosis of this form of dementia seldom survive for more than a year and death usually occurs within months.

Opportunistic infections may also play a role in the development of AIDS-related dementia. One of the most common of these is progressive multifocal leukoencephalopathy which occurs secondarily to infection by another viral agent, the JC virus (a human polyomavirus first isolated in 1971 and named after the initials of the name of the first patient to be discovered with it). Approximately 80% of all individuals carry this virus and in immunocompetent individuals it remains dormant (Moore 2001). However, with the reduced immune function observed in AIDS, the virus becomes active and spreads to the brain where it produces delirium or dementia.

Neuropsychological symptoms

The initial presentation of AD varies greatly from person to person. There are, however, some commonalities. Usually AD has an insidious onset with progressive deterioration and a gradual decline in cognitive abilities, eventually affecting almost all brain functions. Prior to diagnosis, a prodromal phase for the disorder has been proposed in which neuropsychological decline has occurred but the diagnosis of AD has not yet been made (Amieva et al 2005). Studies have suggested that this prodromal phase can last up to 20 years with measurable decline occurring some 2 to 3 years before the manifestation of specific symptoms and some 4 to 5 years before the diagnostic criteria for AD are met (Fox et al 1998).

In the early stages, patients may experience memory impairment, lapses of judgement, and subtle changes in personality. As the disorder progresses, however, these cognitive changes become more pronounced and focal neurological signs become apparent.

Early deficits include poor memory where the patient becomes gradually more and more forgetful with the increasingly rapid loss of newly learned information; for example forgetting the location of keys, the content of a telephone conversation, or what happened earlier in the day. Over time, this anterograde amnesia becomes more outstanding and is often coupled with retrograde amnesia where patients are unable to recall long-stored information such as where they went to school, where they worked, their children's names or if they are/were married.

Often in the early or middle stages of the disorder, this impairment of short-term memory with apparently intact long-term recall can be misleading. Carers, for example, are often confused when the patient appears to be able to recall events clearly from many years previously but are unable to retain more recent information.

Another area of contrast in memory is that episodic rather than procedural memory appears to be affected. Thus, an extremely impaired patient, whilst unable to recall the name of a particular musical instrument, may still be able to play it.

In terms of the behavioural sequelae of these cognitive changes, one might observe an early increased dependence on written notes to aid memory. As the disease progresses and memory becomes ever more impaired there may also be confabulations, an increased frequency of misidentifications and an increased frequency of false recognitions. Finally, there will also be a breakdown of self-awareness with reduced insight and reduced or absent appreciation of the presence of a memory disorder.

Language deficits are also associated with AD and can, again, appear early on in the course of the disease. These include impairments in naming and word retrieval, which often produces ever more circumlocutions in speech, reduced comprehension and reduced verbal fluency. In the late stages of AD, speech becomes extremely impoverished with patients only able to utter simple words or phrases. Eventually, complete mutism ensues.

A similar pattern of language deficits can also be observed in writing skills. Often this dysfunction will become more severe as AD progresses and is further complicated by the influence of other features of the disease that are superimposed upon language functioning. For example, increasing difficulties with praxis will have an inevitable impact on graphomotor skills.

Executive dysfunction also becomes apparent as, even in the early stages, patients typically demonstrate difficulties with the organization, coordination and sequencing of mental activity. The dysfunction is subtle in the early stages of the illness but, as time progresses, the problem becomes more significant as difficulties with abstract reasoning and problem-solving become apparent.

This breakdown of executive skills, then, also has a secondary impact on other cognitive skills, for example memory, as the ability to compensate for dysfunction becomes influenced by poor strategy generation and disorganization. For instance, as mentioned previously, a patient may become more dependent on written notes to aid memory. However, an accompanying executive dysfunction could mean that these notes become scattered or remain unfinished, thus rendering their compensatory value negligible.

Visuospatial dysfunctions also typically become apparent as more substantial degeneration of the parietal and temporal lobes occurs. In day-to-day terms this is often evidenced as problems in orienting in familiar environments. Again, the frequency of these topographical disturbances is correlated with the progression of the disease.

Behaviourally, patients with AD demonstrate a wide variety of symptoms. There are again, however, a number of common factors that can be observed. Often there are agitation, apathy, affective and psychotic symptoms (Mega et al 1996). Personality change can also be observed as an early feature of the disorder, although it is more common for memory problems to be noted as the main presenting factor.

Depressive symptoms are common and range from mild to those associated with major depressive episodes. Anxiety and increased irritability are also found in AD patients, as is the less common euphoria. In addition, both visual and auditory hallucinations can be observed as well as delusions in a proportion of patients.

It is, however, important to remember that at least some of these psychiatric symptoms might be accounted for by way of the cognitive difficulties that the patient experiences. For example, paranoid delusions may be a feature of memory dysfunction, with an accusation of theft made by a patient representing a mechanism for reconciling poor awareness of a memory dysfunction in the case of a mislaid item.

Personality changes can also take many different forms. However, the more common features of this tend to be apathy, indifference and withdrawal (Moore 2001). There may also be increasing impulsiveness, disinhibition and coarseness (Petry et al 1988) and an exaggeration of premorbid personality characteristics.

In summary, during the first stages of AD, memory of recent events, orientation to time and place, attentional skills and spatial perceptions begin to show signs of decline. There may be signs of agitation and fatigue and subtle personality change. Awareness or insight of a memory dysfunction may be limited. In the second stage, the patient will demonstrate a progression of the memory disorder and an increasing problem with judgement, problem-solving and abstract thinking. As the dementia progresses there will be the development of various symptoms suggesting cortical involvement, such as aphasic difficulties, dyspraxia and agnosia, and the development of frontal release signs (reflex behaviours indicating the involvement of the frontal lobes). Finally, in the last stage, there will be a complete failure of intellectual functioning and emotional disinhibition. This may be accompanied by seizures, Kluver-Bucy syndrome, and, very rarely, hemiparesis.

In contrast to AD, the symptom onset in MID is abrupt and, given its aetiological nature, more idiosyncratic. Infarcts in different regions of the cortex and subcortex produce a wide variety of cognitive symptoms; whereas, AD demonstrates a gradual, global decline. In many cases where there has been a large, single infarct or where multiple, smaller infarcts have a more strategic involvement, there may be episodes of apraxia, ataxia and aphasia, followed by periods of recovery. Focal neurological signs may be evident and lateralized neurological deficits such as hemiparesis may also be apparent.

Neuropsychologically, there may be evidence of both anterograde and retrograde amnesia and fluctuating and episodic intellectual decline. There may also be evidence of delusions and hallucinations, depression, and poor emotional control. Nocturnal confusion also appears to be more marked than with AD.

Like AD, LBD is a gradually progressive disorder and shares many of the same neuropsychological symptoms. There are impairments of memory, intellectual and executive functioning, and disturbances of language skills and visuospatial abilities. However, LBD is associated with more marked episodes of confusion, significant fluctuations in cognitive functioning, and research suggests that the attentional, visuoconstructional, visuospatial and psychomotor elements of LBD are greater than those observed in AD (Perry et al 1990).

Also unlike AD, LBD presents in many cases with parkinsonism and has more prominent psychiatric features such as visual hallucinations, paranoid delusions and depression. LBD also shows a greater sensitivity to antipsychotic medication.

FTD stands as distinct from AD in that, while there is an insidious onset, there is degeneration of the frontal and temporal lobes (Neary & Snowden 1996) giving rise early on to the personality changes and problems with adaptive behaviour that precede cognitive impairments. Patients often become apathetic or agitated and restless, there is frequent disinhibition, emotional changes, and social and personal awareness reduction, with a concomitant change in personal hygiene and social behaviour.

Expressive dysphasia is an early feature of this disorder with progression leading to mutism. Judgement and abstract reasoning also become impaired early in the course of the illness while memory functioning remains relatively intact, as do visuospatial and visuoconstructional abilities. Perseveration, planning deficits and cognitive flexibility problems are also observed. Some patients with FTD will demonstrate environmental dependency syndrome and/or Kluver-Bucy syndrome.

HD, being one of the subcortical degenerative diseases, generally presents early on with chorea (irregular and jerky movements outside the patient's control) and/or personality change. Over time and with the progression of the disorder, dementia gradually becomes a feature.

Personality change usually presents as problems with increased irritability, impulsiveness and impairment of judgement. As cognitive problems begin to be observed there are difficulties with attention, memory, calculation, and abstract reasoning. There may also be hallucinations (more often visual than auditory) and paranoid delusions. In contrast to AD, skill learning is generally unimpaired and significant aphasia does not appear to be a common feature. However, visuospatial functions do show signs of deficit.

The executive function deficits observed in HD tend to be similar to those of patients with frontal lobe lesions (Blumer & Benson 1975) and the observed emotional changes suggest that the depression present in many cases of HD might be a result of the disease process rather than a reaction to the illness per se (Lezak 1995).

Another interesting feature of HD appears to be a problem with the identification of the facial expressions of emotion and particularly that of disgust. Research has indicated that even patients who are presymptomatic for the disease appear to be impaired on recognition tasks for a number of emotions (Sprengelmeyer et al 1996) and demonstrate a significant difficulty with the identification of disgust (Gray et al 1997).

The initial presentation of CJD is usually associated with personality change, psychosis, cerebellar symptoms such as ataxia, visual symptoms such as hemianopia, and dementia. As the disorder quickly progresses, almost all cases demonstrate: myoclonus (involuntary contractions of individual muscles or muscle groups); evidence of confusion; and often aphasia, visuospatial impairment, and psychiatric disturbance characterized by hallucinations and delusions and mood changes. A rapid collapse in neurological and neuropsychological functioning ensues and within weeks or months this rapid decline gives way to stupor and coma.

vCJD, on the other hand, generally demonstrates an earlier age onset than CJD but a similar symptom presentation. There are behavioural and personality changes that include insomnia, withdrawal, agitation, and apathy; psychiatric disturbances are evident as depression, emotional lability or psychosis; motor disturbances include ataxia and myoclonus; and there is dementia.

ADC tends to demonstrate a gradual onset and occurs almost exclusively in the later stages of the AIDS illness. The early signs can include apathy, mild memory disorder and attentional problems, and a slowing of both mental and motor functioning. There may also be evidence of emotional changes with mood swings, reduced spontaneity, social withdrawal, increased irritability, emotional lability and depression.

Treatment

Sadly, with the exception of depression and the other causes of reversible dementias mentioned earlier, there are, as yet, no treatments available that halt or reverse the progression of these disorders. Patients, however, may benefit from those treatments that are currently available, including both pharmacological and non-pharmacological therapies.

Many drugs are now available to treat the progressive dementias, and while these do not halt or reverse the cerebral damage caused by a particular disorder, they can improve symptoms and, importantly, slow the progression of the disease. Consequently, such treatments may improve quality of life, ease the burden on carers and delay the need for more intensive care such as admission to a nursing home. It is also true to say that many patients might also benefit from non-pharmacological intervention, particularly in the early stages of the disorder. Such treatments might include cognitive skills training or behaviour modification.

In AD, then, these therapies may be categorized as those that reduce risk, those that retard progression or those that alleviate symptoms (Moore 2001).

Medications that research suggests can reduce the risk of AD include non-steroidal anti-inflammatory drugs or NSAIDs (Aisen & Davis 1994) and oestrogens for post-menopausal women (Tang et al 1996), although it is not yet clear to whom these medications should be given. However, it is thought that those at high risk for the development of AD might be targeted.

In terms of the slowing of progression, vitamin E and, to a lesser degree, the PD medication selegeline (Schneider et al 1993) have been suggested as agents that might slow the progression of AD.

With regard to the pharmacological amelioration of the cognitive symptoms of AD, most of the work done has concentrated on cholinesterase inhibitors. These are drugs that slow the breakdown of the neurotransmitter substance acetylcholine, which is markedly reduced in sufferers of AD. At the time of writing, there are three types of cholinesterase inhibitor licensed in the UK for the treatment of AD. These are donepezil (Aricept), rivastigmine (Exelon) and galantamine (Reminyl). These cholinesterase inhibitors temporarily improve or stabilize cognition in some patients and may help to slow the general decline in mental functions associated with AD.

The use of drug treatments for AD, including the pharmacological management of the other symptoms that can arise from the disorder, such as depression, agitation and psychosis, represents, however, only a small proportion of the possible interventions. Non-pharmacological treatments for AD, and indeed for many of the other dementias, include cognitive skills retraining, reality orientation, validation therapy, reminiscence therapy, and behaviour modification.

Conversely, with regard to the other dementing disorders mentioned here, there are, at present, no specific pharmacological treatments. However, antidepressants and other medications may be useful in the treatment of specific symptoms associated with these diseases.

In MID, for example, there is no standard pharmacological approach. Nevertheless, some of the symptoms arising from the condition will, necessarily, have a common treatment. For instance, selective serotonin reuptake inhibitors (SSRIs) may be prescribed for depression. Almost all other treatments are aimed at reducing the risk of further cerebral damage by CVA. This may involve the prescription of a variety of drugs aimed at diabetes, high cholesterol, or high blood pressure. It might even be the case that agents such as aspirin or warfarin are given to prevent the formation of embolisms or that surgery is recommended to restore the normal blood supply.

To provide a further illustration, in LBD parkinsonism, symptoms may be amenable to levodopa and psychotic symptoms may be open to treatment with neuroleptic medication. However, as mentioned previously, this disorder is extremely sensitive to neuroleptic medication and so care must be taken both to examine the possible use of atypical neuroleptic agents and to look at the interaction of levodopa with these agents.

To conclude, then, in MID, LBD, FTD, HD, CJD, vCJD and AIDS dementia complex (ADC) there is no known treatment that can arrest or reverse degeneration. Current interventions, therefore, are aimed at alleviating presenting symptoms and making the patient as comfortable as possible.

From a neuropsychological perspective, the aim of treatment is usually to accurately assess and monitor functioning and to establish an ongoing relationship with both the patients and their families in order to help them understand and address cognitive and behavioural symptoms. This may also involve rehabilitation of the underlying cognitive deficits with the purpose of slowing progression or maintaining function for as long as possible.

Summary

AD and the other disorders mentioned above, then, demonstrate a variety of pathologies and aetiologies. Each presents with subtle differences in early neuropsychological symptoms and treatments range from the direct, in the case of AD, to the secondary alleviation of difficulties in other conditions. However, the hallmark of these conditions is a progressively debilitating decline in cognitive and behavioural functioning.

CEREBRAL VASCULAR ACCIDENT

Overview

When the blood flow to the brain is disrupted, there is, typically, a rapid presentation of very specific neurological and neuropsychological symptoms, often related to the site where primary disruption has taken place. In the case of very brief interruptions in flow, these symptoms may be transitory. In cases where there is a more significant interruption, symptoms may be more long-lasting, representing structural damage. This section, then, seeks to clarify the mechanisms whereby CVAs occur, the likely symptoms and outcomes, and the potential treatments available.

Description

Cerebral vascular accident (CVA), cerebrovascular event (CVE) or stroke, as it is commonly termed, results from a disruption of the vascular supply to the brain. Once termed apoplexy or an apopleptic attack, CVAs occur either as a consequence of haemorrhage, bleeding from a cerebral artery, or ischaemia, through the occlusion or blockage of a blood vessel.

Commonly, CVA is characterized by the abrupt onset of focal neurological symptoms lasting for more than 24 hours. This focal impairment reflects injury to the areas of the brain supplied by the affected vessel and the location of this damage can be critical in determining initial outcome. For example, a relatively small CVA in the brainstem can cause death, while an equivalent CVA in the right cerebral hemisphere might produce almost no apparent deficit.

The location of the CVA is generally determined by presenting symptoms, since the functional units of the brain supplied by a given vessel will demonstrate a typical general pattern of impairment. For instance, a CVA in the left anterior portion of the brain will usually cause language impairment and contralateral hemiplegia.

Neuroradiological tests such as CT and MRI, during the acute phase of CVA, do not generally demonstrate infarction or tissue death, since there is no immediate change in tissue density. However, CT and MRI do reliably demonstrate haemorrhage, as blood can be visualized in areas that do not usually contain it. Lumbar puncture is also a reliable method in the indication of cerebral haemorrhage in terms of the presence of blood in the CSF.

Epidemiology

CVA is the second largest cause of death worldwide and the largest cause of long-term neurological disability. Mortality rates for CVA, however, have generally declined over the course of the last 50 years (Warlow 1998). Indeed, a more recent study suggests that incidence, as a whole, has fallen by up to 40% in the UK during the past 20 years, notwithstanding an increase in the population of individuals aged 75 years and over (Rothwell et al 2004).

Despite these trends, however, a brief examination of the statistics for CVA offers a sobering reminder of its impact. To illustrate, around 130 000 people in England and Wales suffer a CVA annually, with some 68 000 deaths occurring as a result of CVA annually; it is the third most common cause of death in England and Wales, after heart disease and cancer (Warlow et al 1996). Of these cases, around 85% are the result of a cerebral infarction, while 15% are the result of cerebral haemorrhage (Ballinger & Patchett 2004).

The incidence of CVA, as might be expected, increases with age (Hachinsky & Norris 1985) and is uncommon under the age of 40 years (Ballinger & Patchett 2004). It is slightly more common in men than in woman (Kurtzke 1983).

Pathology

To understand the pathology of CVAs, one must first appreciate something of the brain's blood supply. Blood is supplied to the brain by three major artery systems: the right and left internal carotid arteries, and the vertebral/basilar system (Fig. 6.1). The carotid arteries supply the more anterior portions of the cerebral hemispheres and the vertebral/basilar system supplies both the posterior portions of the cerebral hemispheres and the brainstem and cerebellum.

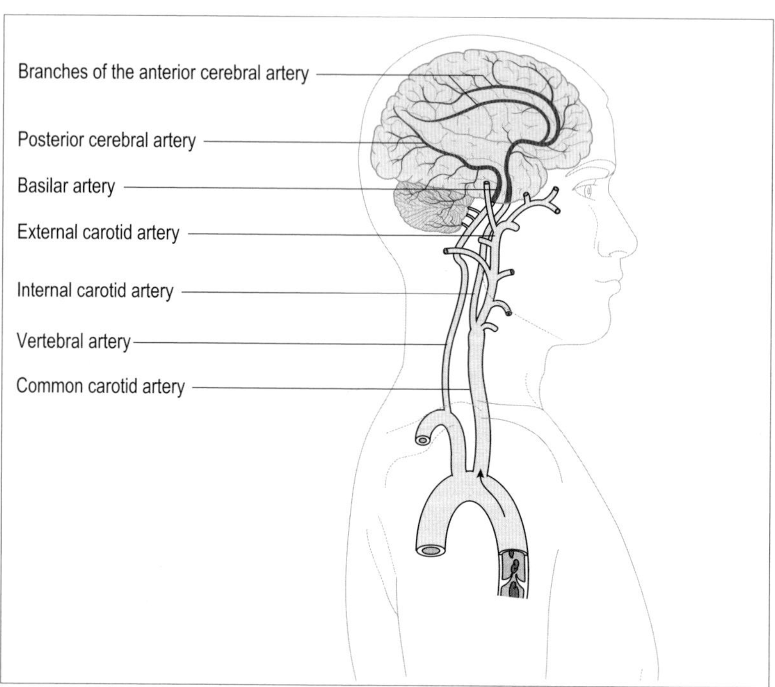

Fig. 6.1 Brain arterial supply. (After Smart 2001)

As the internal carotid arteries ascend through each hemisphere, they divide or bifurcate into two branches: the anterior and middle cerebral arteries. The anterior cerebral artery supplies the inferior surface of the frontal lobe and the medial parts of the hemisphere, while the middle cerebral artery supplies the basal ganglia, deep white matter of the brain and the lateral surface of the hemisphere.

The vertebral arteries, on the other hand, run upward through the cervical vertebrae of the neck and enter the base of the skull through the foramen magnum. The two vertebral arteries then join and form the basilar artery. This artery supplies the pons, cerebellum and midbrain. As the basilar artery reaches the top of the cerebellum it bifurcates to form the two posterior cerebral arteries. These posterior cerebral arteries supply the thalamus, the medial surface of the temporal lobes and the occipital lobes.

The venous flow of deoxygenated blood from the brain drains through the superficial veins on the surface of the cerebral hemispheres, and ultimately into the superior sagittal sinus. The brain's deep structures and its inferior surface are served by a system that eventually forms the straight sinus. These two sinuses in the posterior portion of the brain ultimately form the jugular veins in the neck.

With this basic knowledge of the vascular system in mind, then, we can appreciate that the nature and extent of the neurological and neuropsychological deficits observed will depend on the arterial vessel involved. However, we still need to differentiate the mechanism of damage. As mentioned above, there are basically two types of CVA: ischaemic and haemorrhagic.

Ischaemic CVAs result from a drop in blood pressure sufficient to deprive the tissues of glucose (ischaemia) and oxygen (anoxia). The consequence of such changes is the death of cells and atrophy of brain tissue over a period of days. This is referred to as cerebral infarction. By far the most common forms of ischaemic CVAs are the result of atherosclerosis, thrombosis and embolism.

In atherosclerosis, lipid deposits in the form of plaques line the artery walls and build up over the course of time. This build up may eventually reduce arterial flow, completely block the artery, or produce an embolus that flows in the arterial stream to block the artery further in its course. Thrombosis or the formation of a blood clot around an atherosclerotic plaque or an embolism produced by, for example, cardiac disease, may have the same effect, although peculiarly, embolisms appear to most often affect the middle cerebral artery on the left side of the brain.

However, whatever the mechanism, if a vessel becomes occluded, the tissues supplied by that artery no longer receive the necessary nutrients and oxygen and the tissues eventually die: an infarction.

Transient ischaemic attacks (TIAs) result from a reduced flow of blood to the brain in the early stages of vascular damage. Generally, the focal neurological signs associated with such TIAs are sudden in onset but relatively short lived. That is to say, they can last for minutes or hours, sometimes as long as 24 hours. The temporary impairments observed in TIAs are typically the result of brief interruption of the blood flow in the carotid or vertebral/basilar arterial systems and are a warning that a patient may suffer a later CVA.

Haemorrhagic CVAs, on the other hand, result from bleeding into the brain tissues producing damage by mass effect, infarction, and direct destruction of nervous tissue by the blood. Certain areas of the brain also appear to be at greater risk than others, notably the pons, cerebellum, thalamus and basal ganglia. The most frequent cause of such a cerebral haemorrhage is hypertension, high blood pressure, while the most common structural cause is the presence of a cerebral aneurysm.

Intracerebral haemorrhage, a bleeding into the tissues of the brain, is most commonly caused by hypertension where sustained elevations of blood pressure result in progressive weakening of the walls of small arteries. This process of deterioration may result in the development of small haemorrhages and infarction known as lacunar infarcts. Alternatively, the patient may develop an aneurysm and, eventually, a larger haemorrhage. A large proportion of patients suffering an intracerebral haemorrhage will die as the release of blood from a ruptured vessel under arterial pressure can cause extensive damage to the brain.

Subarachnoid haemorrhage typically occurs as a result of the rupture of an aneurysm in an artery at the base of the brain. Blood from this rupture is dispersed in the subarachnoid space and results in an increase in intracranial pressure.

Another cause of both intracerebral and subarachnoid haemorrhages are arteriovenous malformations (AVMs). These congenital abnormalities represent malfunctioning communication between arteries, capillaries and veins. AVMs exist as a mass of thin-walled vessels which may be predisposed to rupture, causing haemorrhage. AVMs may also cause seizures and headache.

Finally, silent strokes are CVAs that demonstrate no obvious neurological symptoms. These tend to be associated with small lacunar infarcts. They do not usually become apparent until a patient is investigated with CT or MRI for other reasons, when a more obvious or serious CVA occurs, or when behavioural changes take place.

Aetiology

The wide range of disorders having an influence on cerebral circulation is, obviously, beyond the scope of this book. However, the various risk factors for CVA are fairly well known and so an examination of these factors is considered useful.

Risk factors are individual characteristics or behaviours that increase the risk of disease. Some of those associated with CVA can be treated or controlled; other factors, however, cannot. Naturally, the more presenting factors an individual has, the greater their risk of CVA. Amongst the factors that can be controlled or treated are hypertension, smoking, diabetes mellitus, carotid artery disease, peripheral artery disease, cardiovascular disease, blood disorders such as high normal haemoglobin concentration and sickle cell anaemia, high levels of cholesterol, oestrogen containing oral contraceptives, physical inactivity and obesity, excessive alcohol use, and the use of illicit intoxicants such as cocaine.

Amongst the factors that cannot be modified by treatment are increasing age, gender (CVA is more common in men than in women), a family history of CVA, and a previous history of CVA or heart attack.

Neuropsychological symptoms

As might be expected, the neuropsychological presentation of symptoms in cases of CVA varies greatly. Impairment in any cognitive skill can be observed. This, however, is determined by the arterial vessel or vessels involved, the severity of the CVA and, to some degree, the period of time that causative factors have had an influence before the CVA. What follows, then, is a brief and far from exhaustive description of the more common general deficits associated with CVA and also an appreciation of the implications for the involvement of the specific areas supplied by particular arterial vessels.

Most commonly, in patients where the CVA involves the cerebral hemisphere dominant for language (usually the left hemisphere), there is an associated disturbance of language functioning giving rise to aphasia. In the limbs contralateral to the CVA, it is often the case that motor deficits can be observed. In more severe cases this can be observed as hemiplegia.

Typically, damage to the right cerebral hemisphere causes a perceptual deficit and often a left sided hemi-neglect causing the patient to ignore the left side of space. The opposite of this can be seen, although more rarely, in cases of left cerebral hemisphere CVA and right-sided hemi-neglect.

Such general observations are useful as far as they go. However, they do not provide an illustration of the spectrum of neuropsychological symptoms associated with CVA. Nor do they help us localize the damage done. In order to get a more detailed picture, then, it is necessary to look in more detail at the specific vessels involved and the deficits that might arise from their involvement.

The basilar artery (BA) supplies blood to the brain stem and medulla, dividing ultimately into the posterior cerebral arteries. Incomplete occlusion of this vessel can lead to vertigo, ataxia, paresis, sensory loss and paraesthesia. At its most extreme, occlusion of certain of the BAs branch vessels can lead to locked-in syndrome, where the patient is paralyzed and unable to communicate with the outside world except through some retained eye movements.

In very rare cases of CVA involving branches of the BA, there can be strategic damage to the medulla resulting in Ondine's curse, a loss of the involuntary control of breathing (Ondine was a nymph from Greek mythology cursed by Zeus to think about every breath she took). Thus, while voluntary control remains unimpaired (e.g. one can consciously control the lungs in order to hold a breath, exhale, or hyperventilate) unconscious or involuntary control is lost or impaired. In very simple terms, the patient simply forgets to breath.

The posterior cerebral artery (PCA), arising from the basilar artery, supplies blood to the occipital lobes, parts of the temporal lobes and the thalamus. Occlusions to this vessel, therefore, most commonly result in visual field deficits, Anton's syndrome, and prosopagnosia.

Infarcts involving the PCA and the primary cerebral hemisphere (again usually the left cerebral hemisphere) often lead to impairments of memory, difficulty with reading skills, and a type of aphasia producing problems with the comprehension of language but at the same time having no influence on the patient's own speech. On the other hand, PCA involvement in the non-dominant cerebral hemisphere (usually the right cerebral hemisphere) can lead to a reduced awareness of sensory information from the opposite side of the body.

The internal carotid artery (ICA) branches to form the anterior and middle cerebral arteries and supplies blood to the more anterior and medial structures of the brain. Occlusion in this vessel can result in ipsilateral blindness, contralateral hemiplegia, and aphasia. TIAs associated with the ICA can result in temporary, monocular blindness (amaurosis fugax – fleeting blindness), paraesthesia, aphasia and contralateral hemiparesis.

The anterior cerebral artery (ACA) is a branch of the internal carotid artery lying above the optic nerve and following the line of the corpus callosum. It supplies blood to the frontal and parietal lobes as well as the corpus callosum. Damage to the supplied areas can result in contralateral motor impairments. Unilateral damage to the dominant cerebral hemisphere often results in aphasia and deficits in voluntary movement, while bilateral frontal lobe infarction can result in akinetic mutism.

The middle cerebral artery (MCA) is the largest branch of the internal carotid artery and supplies blood to anterior and medial portions of the cortex and, therefore, to the frontal, temporal and parietal lobes. Occlusion involving this vessel may produce contralateral hemiplegia and/or contralateral hemianaesthesia. If the dominant hemisphere is affected there may also be aphasia, left-right disorientation and reduced arithmetic ability.

Treatment

The medical treatment of CVAs is to some degree limited and, therefore, usually supportive. Treatment is undertaken primarily to prevent complications, limit the damage done and minimize disability. Most patients make considerable recovery after 6 months following onset with the bulk of recovery having taken place within the first 2 years. As regards outcome indicators, death or long-term disability has been found to be correlated with urinary incontinence (Skilbeck 2003).

Drug treatments are aimed at dealing with the effects of CVAs, the prevention of complications, and a reduction in the risk of further CVAs. Of the many pharmacological treatments, the more common are antiplatelet drug agents such as aspirin, anticoagulants such as heparin or warfarin, and antihypertensives to reduce blood pressure.

Surgically, carotid endarterectomy is used to clear the arteries of atherosclerotic plaques and may be used to treat partial occlusion of carotid arteries resulting in TIAs. The surgical evacuation of a haemorrhage is also a common treatment following this type of CVA, while the resection of aneurysms or AV malformations may also be possible if these defects are accessible.

However, despite these various treatments, almost half of those that survive a CVA will be left with significant disability. Nevertheless, the brain is remarkably adaptable and in the time after a CVA, many of the tissues that have sustained damage are able to recover some of their function. In concert with this recovery of function, other brain areas are able to compensate for some of those functions demonstrating impairment. Perhaps the most important aspect of CVA treatment, therefore, is rehabilitation.

The general aim of rehabilitation, therefore, is to stimulate and enhance the process of recovery and adaptation, and an intensive programme after CVA is likely to involve a multidisciplinary team including physicians, physiotherapists, speech and language therapists, occupational therapists and neuropsychologists. Starting this programme early in the course of the illness can substantially improve recovery and reduce the effects of disability.

The rehabilitation process is, of course, tailored to meet the needs of individual patients but may include: medical support in order to prevent potential medical or psychological complications; cognitive retraining; support to aid in physical recovery; assistance in the management of the physical, emotional and social effects of the CVA, and the provision of aids to encourage the patient to become as independent as possible.

Summary

CVA occurs when there is a disruption of the vascular supply to the brain resulting from haemorrhage, ischaemia or occlusion. There is usually a rapid onset of focal symptoms related to the location of the vascular event. The history in each case often highlights a number of pre-existing risk factors, some of which represent aspects of lifestyle which can be modified, and some of which represent aetiological factors that are more fixed and cannot be changed. Individual neuropsychological symptoms vary greatly. These tend, however, to be closely linked to the site and severity of the CVA. Treatment is usually aimed at the prevention of complications and the reduction of risk for further CVAs. Nevertheless, a great number of those suffering a CVA will be left with residual disability. Compensatory techniques and rehabilitation interventions are, therefore, essential to returning patients to as independent a lifestyle as possible.

EPILEPSY

Overview

A seizure represents a transient abnormal electrical discharge within the cells of the brain. The continuing tendency towards these seizures is termed epilepsy. Such seizures can result in a complex array of behavioural and cognitive symptoms. This section on epileptic phenomena aims to increase the reader's understanding of the variety of presentations and neuropsychological disturbances that can occur and some of the treatments which can be applied.

Description

A seizure or ictus is an abrupt onset episode resulting from abnormal electrical discharges in cerebral neurons producing changes in behaviour and/or levels of consciousness. There are, of course, many different causes of seizure; for example hypocalcaemia and alcohol withdrawal. The term epilepsy, however, is generally reserved for those cases where there has been more than one seizure and the suggestion is that the causes of the seizures would, if untreated, give rise to further episodes.

Usually associated with recurrent convulsive episodes, the term epilepsy is actually used to describe any repeated paroxysmal event from the more familiar grand mal/tonic-clonic seizures to the more subtle manifestations represented by simple partial seizures. In short, the variety of presentation is extremely varied, reflecting the involvement of the cerebral system or systems. Seizures may cause abnormal actions, complex motor disturbances, perceptual phenomena, sensory experiences, mood fluctuations, behavioural and cognitive changes and may even affect the way an individual grasps reality, such is the singular and idiosyncratic nature of the dysfunctions associated with these ictal events.

Broadly, epilepsy is classified according to the symptoms and signs of the seizures, rather than the presence of specific aetiological factors. As a result, not surprisingly, there are many different types of seizure. Box 6.1 provides an abbreviated list of epilepsy classifications derived from the International Classification of Epileptic Seizures (Commission on Classification and Terminology of the International League Against Epilepsy 1981). In general, however, one may differentiate between generalized and partial seizures, the latter accounting for approximately 80% of all adult epilepsies (Fig. 6.2).

Simple partial seizures are those that appear to have a local onset within the brain but have no effect on consciousness. They are typically short-lived and present as motor, sensory, autonomic or psychic types. The motor type is characterized by disturbance of the motor cortex of the brain and produces symptoms such as involuntary movement, paralysis, or, if the disturbance spreads through the motor cortex, a wave of involuntary movement starting, for example in a finger, and then extending to the hand, then the arm, the shoulder and face. This is termed the Jacksonian March or a Jacksonian seizure after the English 19th Century neurologist John Hughlings Jackson.

Sensory types can produce either positive or negative somatosensory sensations such as tingling, numbness or pain, while those that affect the special senses can produce simple visual, auditory, olfactory or gustatory hallucinations.

Autonomic varieties, on the other hand, often produce nausea, vomiting, pallor or sweating. Finally, there are those simple seizures that produce psychic phenomena such as cognitive disturbances or emotional/mood changes including déjà vu feelings, depersonalization, anxiety, depression, or sometimes euphoria.

Complex partial seizures, again, demonstrate an apparently local onset and are most frequently associated with the temporal lobe, giving rise to the term temporal lobe epilepsy (TLE). Complex partial seizures are character-

Box 6.1 Epilepsy classification

(Adapted from the International Classification of Epileptic Seizures)

1. Partial seizures
Those seizures that appear to begin locally and then spread, reflecting a small local electrical disturbance. These can be further subdivided into:

(a) *Simple seizures (without loss of consciousness)*: motor, sensory (either somato or special sensory), autonomic, and/or psychic symptoms
(b) *Complex seizures (with impaired consciousness)*: beginning as simple partial seizures and progressing to impairment of consciousness or with impaired consciousness at the outset
(c) *Partial seizures developing to secondarily generalized seizures*: simple partial seizures evolving to generalized seizures, complex partial seizures developing into generalized seizures, or simple partial seizures that evolve into complex partial seizures that become generalized.

2. Generalized seizures
These seizures may be convulsive or non-convulsive and appear bilaterally without apparent local onset. They can be further subdivided into:

(a) *Absence seizures (petit mal)*: producing an impairment of consciousness only, with tonic components, with atonic components, autonomic components, and/or automatisms and with the exception of impairment of consciousness, appearing either alone or in combination
(b) *Myoclonic seizures*
(c) *Clonic seizures*
(d) *Tonic seizures*
(e) *Tonic-clonic seizures (grand mal)*
(f) *Atonic seizures*

3. Other unclassified seizures
This category contains a number of groups which remain, owing to a lack of data, generally unclassified. Examples include musicogenic epilepsy where certain tones or musical themes prompt a seizure, and arithmetical epilepsy where performing calculations prompts a seizure.

ized by a disturbance of consciousness, can last for anywhere between one and several minutes and can be preceded by an aura (itself a simple partial seizure, producing the subjective experiences preceding the onset of a more complex seizure).

Typically, the only behavioural symptom of such a seizure is automatism. Automatisms are purposeless, simple, repetitive movements. These can include simple scratching, swallowing, blinking, lip smacking or chewing, etc., or more complex behaviours such as walking or running. Usually, the disturbance of consciousness is associated with a disruption of continuous memory. Commonly, the sufferer in the post-ictal or post seizure phase complains of headache and confusion.

Simple partial and complex partial seizures may also secondarily generalize into generalized seizures. Generalized seizures can thus be seen as primary or secondary, arising in the absence of a partial seizure or secondary

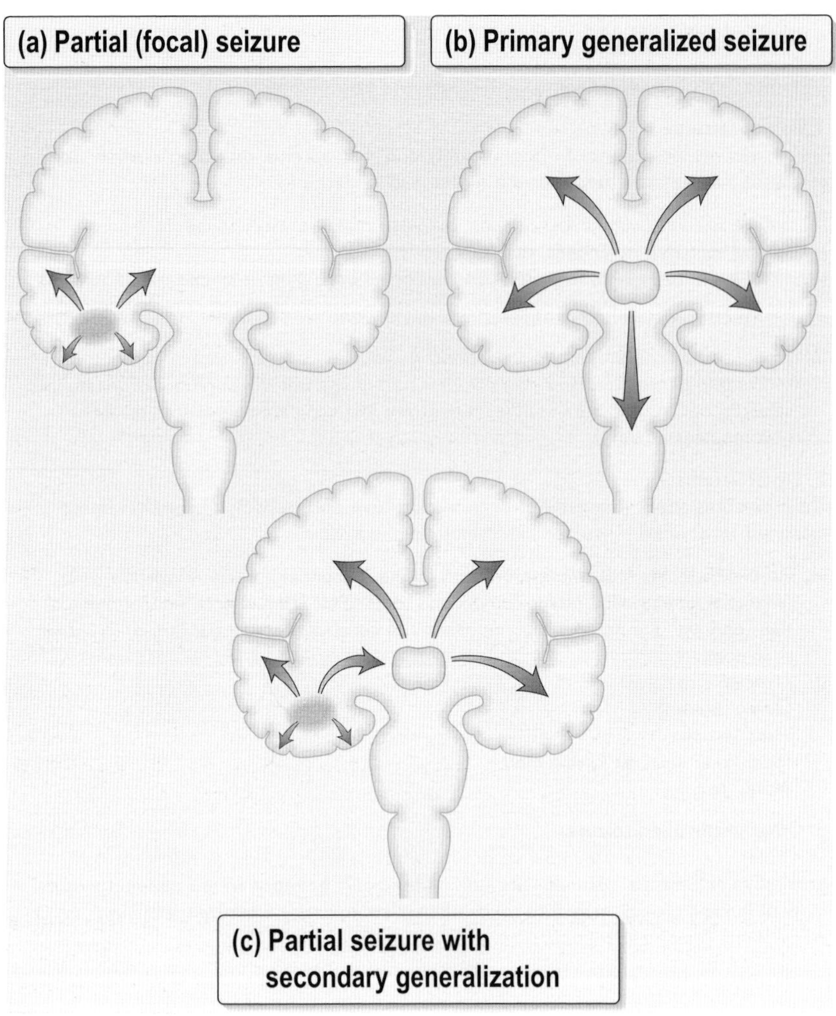

Fig. 6.2 Basic seizure types. (From Kumar & Clark 2005)

to a partial seizure. Generalized seizures arise from subcortical structures and involve both hemispheres of the brain. Unlike partial seizures, they appear to have no local onset and can be either convulsive or non-convulsive.

Absence seizures (petit mals) are non-convulsive but accompanied by a brief alteration in level of consciousness giving rise to a vacant stare and sometimes this is accompanied by myoclonic jerks. The sufferer maintains muscle tone and bladder control but mental and physical activity become disrupted. Symptoms may last for between 5 and 15 seconds and can occur frequently throughout the day. Often such brief changes can be overlooked by the untrained or inexperienced observer. Usually, absence seizures occur in childhood and only rarely persist into adulthood.

Generalized convulsive seizures come in a number of forms. Until recently, all convulsive seizures came under the heading of grand mal seizures. However, this term is now reserved for the most frequently encountered form, the tonic-clonic seizure characterized by a loss of consciousness and flexion then extension of the muscles. Often there is loss of bladder and/or bowel control, there may be tongue biting and, at the start of the seizure, the sufferer may cry out, an action caused by the tonic contraction of the respiratory muscles.

As regards the other forms, myoclonic seizures give rise to sudden but brief muscular contractions and jerks in the limbs, often occurring in the morning within a short time of waking up. Clonic seizures, by contrast, are characterized by repetitive jerking over the entire body, while tonic seizures are associated with a rigid muscular contraction. Atonic seizures, also known as drop attacks, involve a sudden loss of muscle tone, causing the sufferer to fall.

Finally, we come to status epilepticus, a potentially life threatening condition where the sufferer experiences repeated seizures without fully recovering. Usually, status epilepticus is said to be present when the patient has either had a single prolonged seizure or multiple seizures with no opportunity for recovery between them for a period of 30 minutes (Moore 2001).

Status epilepticus can occur with both partial and generalized seizures. In the former case the varieties include simple partial status (also referred to as epilepsia partialis continua) and complex partial status (also referred to as psychomotor status); in the latter the most dramatic and life-threatening form is that associated with grand mal/tonic-clonic seizures.

Epidemiology

Epilepsy is considered to be a common neurological disorder (Cull & Goldstein 1997). According to the National Society for Epilepsy, at least 300 000 people in the UK have epilepsy and there are some 40 million sufferers worldwide. Research indicates a rate of approximately 4–7 cases per 1000 of the population in adults (Hauser & Annegers 1993) making this the second most common neurological disorder (Adams & Victor 1993).

While everyone has the potential to have an epileptic seizure and 5% of the population will suffer a single seizure at some time in their lives (Lindsay et al 1997), recurrent epileptic seizures usually present first in childhood or adolescence, or in elderly populations, although they can occur at any time. According to the British Epilepsy Association there is a slight difference between the sexes, suggesting a slightly higher rate for males than females. However, while this difference is found consistently, such observations fail to reach statistical significance (Hauser & Annegers 1993).

Of the 0.5% of the population that have recurrent seizures, 70% of these are well controlled with treatment, while the remaining 30% are at least partially resistant to treatment (Lindsay et al 1997). As regards the prevalence rates for each of the subcategories of epilepsy, variations in the diagnosis and clinical definition of seizure type has resulted in difficulties in determining accurate statistics. However, there have been some attempts to analyze rates by seizure type, one such estimate suggesting that 62% of cases are associated with a partial onset, while the remaining 38% of cases represent primary generalized seizures (Lechtenberg 1990).

Unsurprisingly, epilepsy is also associated with an increased risk of mortality, both primarily and secondarily. For example, in the UK, epilepsy-related deaths in young adults are three times higher than the norm, while the highest risk group is young males, aged between 20 years and 30 years, with a history of uncontrolled epilepsy and who experience tonic-clonic seizures.

An increased risk of mortality in these cases may be related to: the aetiological components of the seizures such as a tumour or cerebral infection; the secondary effects of the environmental circumstances of the seizures, such as drowning, suffering burns, or experiencing a head injury; secondary physiological factors, such as cardiopulmonary arrest during a seizure; the considerable physiological impact of status epilepticus; or suicide.

Pathology

Epileptic seizures can originate from anywhere in the brain, both cortically and subcortically (Stevenson & King 1987). In many cases these recurrent seizures are associated with the pathological changes that occur secondarily to other disorders such as CVA, traumatic brain injury, and neurodegenerative illness, etc. When there is a known cause, the condition is termed symptomatic epilepsy. The reader is, therefore, directed to the relevant pathology sections under each of these subheadings.

In as many as two-thirds of all cases, however, no specific cause can be identified (Lishman 1987). In these cases of what is termed idiopathic epilepsy, it is assumed that the patient is possessed of a low convulsive threshold through the inhibition of the neurotransmitter gamma-aminobutyric acid (GABA), causing excessive excitation within the brain (Rankin et al 1996).

Finally, in some cases where there is no clear symptomatic or idiopathic pattern, a diagnosis of cryptogenic epilepsy might be made. This suggests that, although a specific cause cannot be isolated and a low seizure threshold is not thought to be a factor, a physical origin for the seizures is suspected.

Aetiology

The causes of epilepsy are numerous. Box 6.2 shows a far from exhaustive list of the various aetiologies associated with seizures. In cases of symptomatic epilepsy, the aetiological precipitants may be quite clear. For example, post-traumatic epilepsy may develop after a severe head injury. In cryptogenic cases and idiopathic cases the aetiology is far from clear and in many cases a cause for the onset of seizures may never be found.

In addition to the causes listed in Box 6.2 the role of genetics has also been investigated with regard to epilepsy, with current research suggesting a large genetic component (Kaneko et al 2002). However, while some studies have isolated some specific syndromes, such as autosomal dominant nocturnal frontal lobe epilepsy (Hirose et al 1999), the multifactorial nature of the disorder has made studies into this area extremely difficult.

Box 6.2 The causes of seizure

External causation
Traumatic brain injury
Cerebrovascular accident
Intoxicant abuse
Alcohol withdrawal
Medications

Congenital disorders
Down's syndrome
Fragile X syndrome
Autism
Klinefelter's syndrome
Cerebral palsy
Tuberous sclerosis

Neurodegenerative disorders
Alzheimer's disease
Multi-infarct dementia
AIDS dementia
Creutzfeld-Jakob disease
Wilson's disease

Metabolic disorders
Hyperglycaemia
Hypoglycaemia
Hypocalcaemia
Hyponatraemia

Infectious processes
Viral meningitis
Bacterial meningitis
Neurosyphilis

Miscellaneous causes
Tumour
Vascular malformations
Migraine
Vascular disease

To illustrate, a great deal of the work in this field has focused on the difference between primary and secondary expressions of genetic disorder; that is, seizures that may be principally related to a genetic defect and those that are secondarily related to other neurological disorders (Engel 1989). For example, a primary genetic expression would include autosomal dominant lateral temporal epilepsy (Poza et al 1999) where a specific genetic mechanism is isolated. Conversely, neurofibromatosis would be classified as a secondary cause, as the condition is inherited with seizures occurring as a result.

Obviously, a detailed examination of the genetic influences on epilepsy is beyond the scope of this book. However, if one excludes those cases where seizures are symptomatic of another disorder, it is generally thought that the lowered seizure threshold of idiopathic epilepsy may be inherited. Other observations of epilepsy populations have also suggested that the risk of seizure development is lower if only one parent is affected by epilepsy, that the risk of inheritance of absence seizures is greater than for that of partial or other generalized epilepsies, but that the risk is generally higher for the inheritance of generalized idiopathic epilepsy than for partial epilepsy.

Neuropsychological symptoms

As might be expected of a disorder that can originate virtually anywhere in the brain, there is no characteristic pattern of neuropsychological dysfunction in epilepsy. However, the majority of epilepsy sufferers are well controlled with treatment and will not demonstrate significant cognitive difficulties. There are, however, a number of deficits that can be generally observed in those cases where more problematic epilepsy is encountered. It is important, therefore, to distinguish between those impairments that are temporary and linked primarily to the seizure itself, those that represent a lasting, inter-ictal disturbance, and those that might represent the underlying pathology of other conditions producing epilepsy.

In general terms, patients with greater abnormalities observed on EEG traces demonstrate a greater reduction in overall levels of functioning, reflecting a higher level of cerebral involvement in symptomatic epilepsy. Similarly, patients with generalized seizures tend to demonstrate a greater degree of disturbance than do patients with focal seizures and there may also be a further decline observed with increasing seizure frequency.

In terms of the disturbances associated with the ictus itself, these tend to be modified by the nature and site of the disturbance but are generally short lived, depending on the individual's post-ictal recovery. Obviously, the deficits associated with seizures disrupting consciousness will be global. In other types of seizure, the disturbance of cognition is typically associated with the structures involved. Brief cognitive disturbance may be observed in patients experiencing momentary epileptic discharges within the brain. Often these transient disturbances reflect the origin of the discharge. For example, disturbances involving the left hemisphere of the brain might briefly impair verbal functions.

With more obvious seizure activity, less subtle changes in cognition may be noted. For example, patients who suffer an amnestic seizure, with no apparent disturbance of consciousness, will demonstrate a significant if brief disturbance of memory. In these cases, there may be both anterograde or retrograde amnesia or both. To illustrate, a patient might recall events that lead up to seizure onset and behave normally during the seizure itself. However, they will have no recall of events taking place during the seizure (Palmini et al 1992).

In more serious cases, however, where the seizure is prolonged, patients might present with more serious neuropsychological deficits. Non-convulsive status epilepticus, for example, can produce a general disturbance that is similar to that seen in dementia. These symptoms, fortunately, dissipate with time and treatment.

As regards the more persistent, inter-ictal cognitive disturbances, these are usually associated with underlying aetiology. Dysfunctions of attentional, language, memory, and executive functions have all been associated with epilepsy. Memory disturbance, for example, is common amongst epilepsy patients (Trimble & Thompson 1986). However, memory impairments are most common in cases of TLE, with many patients demonstrating a specific deficit for either verbal or non-verbal material depending on the lateralization of the epileptic focus and with bilateral involvement of the temporal lobes producing the most severe impairments.

Emotional and behavioural disturbances have also been associated with epilepsy and occur more frequently with epilepsy than in the general population (Lezak 1995). However, it is again important to remember that it is likely that these disturbances may reflect both the numerous negative aspects of suffering from a neurological disorder as well as a manifestation of cerebral pathology. For instance, a patient's anxious or depressive reaction to seizures might represent the unpredictable or embarrassing nature of these paroxysmal events rather than a pre-ictal sign of simple partial seizure.

That said, some patients with TLE have been reported as tending towards unpleasant personality characteristics (Bear et al 1982). These include humourlessness, obsessionality, irritability, verbosity, hypergraphia, hyper-religiosity, outbursts of anger, and a quality referred to as viscosity, relating to a set of interpersonal characteristics including an over-attention to detail, protracted expressive speech and response style, and difficulty in separating from individuals or terminating conversations, etc. In addition, psychosis has also been observed in some cases of epilepsy as both an ictal and inter-ictal phenomenon (Thompson & Shorvon 1997), while instances of aggression, although rare, have also been reported (Pincus & Tucker 1985). This latter observation, however, is typically associated with an ictal response to external restraint.

Treatment

There are a number of different ways in which epilepsy can be treated. These include the use of medication, surgery, the ketogenic diet, psychological intervention, and the avoidance of seizure triggers.

Medication is the main method used in the management of seizures. However, the use of such medications can produce a number of unwanted side-effects. These include lethargy, tiredness, weight gain, skin rash and dizziness. It is also important to remember that anti-epileptic medications can also be the cause of cognitive impairments through their action to reduce excitability within the cells and can, if not properly monitored, lead to toxicity. Box 6.3 provides a list of the most common anti-epileptic medications.

Box 6.3 Common anticonvulsant (anti-epileptic) medications

Generic name	Brand name
Carbamazepine	Tegretol
Clobazam	–
Clonazepam	Rivotril
Ethosuximide	Zarontin
Gabapentin	Neurontin
Lamotrigine	Lamictal
Levetiracetam	Keppra
Oxcarbazepine	Trileptal
Phenobarbitol	–
Phenytoin	Epanutin
Primidone	Mysoline
Sodium valproate	Epilim
Tiagabine	Gabitril
Topiramate	Topamax
Vigabatrin	Sabril

Importantly, the use of anti-epileptic drugs during pregnancy can interfere with the formation of the nervous system and specifically the formation of the neural tube from which the brain and spinal cord develop. This can, of course, lead to birth defects.

In patients with particularly complex epilepsy, treatment with medication may not prevent recurrent seizures. In these cases a number of surgical procedures can be utilized to remove the epileptic focus and prevent generalization of a seizure, provided that the seizures arise from a single focus within the brain.

Hemispherectomy is performed in those with major, extensive damage to an entire hemisphere of the brain. In children the hemisphere that remains takes over some of the functions of the removed hemisphere. However, there are lasting effects from this type of surgery including weakness and loss of some movement in the contralateral side of the body.

Lobectomy involves the total or partial removal of a single lobe of the brain, the most common form being the removal of the anterior temporal lobe. Corpus callostomies, on the other hand, prevent the spread of seizure activity between the hemispheres by way of a section of corpus callosum. Multiple subpial transections, meanwhile, involve the isolation of an epileptic focus from surrounding tissues preventing the spread of the seizure. This type of procedure is performed when regions important for cognition are involved.

A more recent development that also involves surgical intervention is vagus nerve stimulation. This involves the implanting of a programmable nerve stimulator under the skin with electrodes connected to the vagus nerve in the neck. The device is then programmed to deliver short bursts of electrical energy to the brain via the vagus nerve. Unfortunately, although an improvement has been reported with this procedure, complete seizure control is rare.

The ketogenic diet is a medically supervised diet plan high in fat and low in protein and carbohydrates. The diet is thought to work by promoting the production of excess ketones. It appears to be most effective in children, but may not be tolerated because the diet is considered unpalatable.

Neuropsychological interventions can also prove useful in certain cases of epilepsy by providing a means of formal cognitive assessment as well as a route for support and, importantly, education. In addition, the neuropsychologist may be best placed to offer other inputs such as biofeedback training and relaxation training, particularly when stress is viewed as an epileptogenic.

Finally, triggering events for reflex seizures are also an important causative factor, even though the specific underlying aetiology may be unknown, as these may offer a means of seizure reduction by avoiding the precipitant. It is sometimes useful, therefore, to ask patients to maintain a record of seizures in order that any patterns may be elucidated.

Summary

Occurring as a result of abnormal electrical discharges within cerebral neurons, a seizure is a paroxysmal event often producing changes in consciousness, behaviour and cognition. The focus for these abnormal discharges and the presentation vary from case to case. Generally speaking, however, there is a correlation between the presenting symptoms and the site of the event within the brain. Classification, therefore, of the different types of seizure is according to the signs and symptoms presented. Seizures can originate anywhere within the brain. Sometimes these events are associated with obviously aetiological components such as structural brain damage. In the great majority of cases, however, seizures occur without a known cause. Treatment is usually by way of medication. However, in certain cases, surgical, dietary and psychological treatments may also be offered as an adjunct.

MULTIPLE SCLEROSIS

Overview

Multiple sclerosis is an unpredictable inflammatory disorder causing a constellation of neurological and neuropsychological symptoms. The nature of the condition is such that there is a great deal of variance in presentation and early diagnosis can sometimes prove difficult. In many cases there is relapse and remission; in others there is a rapid progression of symptomatology. Here, we will try to disentangle some of the components of this disorder with a view to clarifying what is known about the pathophysiology and understanding the link between this and the variety of neuropsychological presentations.

Description

First recognized in the 19th Century by the British pathologist Robert Carswell and later detailed by the French neurologist Jean-Martin Charcot, multiple sclerosis (MS) is an inflammatory condition involving the CNS. Normally, this involvement includes the periventricular regions of the brain, the optic nerves, brainstem, cerebellum and spinal cord. This results in motor, visual, balance, sensation and neuropsychological disturbances.

In those affected by MS, this inflammatory process causes damage to the insulating sheath covering the nerve fibre. This insulating layer, called myelin, is produced by oligodendrocytes, a type of glial cell, and its loss, demyelination, results in a disruption of normal nervous impulses. The neuropathological marker for MS, then, is the plaque that indicates damage to the myelin surrounding nerve fibres. In plaques that are active, inflammation and demyelination can be observed, while older plaques that do not appear to be active are observed to be sclerotic or scarred.

In general, because of the great variability in the site or sites affected by demyelination and the differing degrees of severity, MS presents differently in different individuals. It can, therefore, be extremely difficult to diagnose and predict. Typically, however, MS follows one of four possible courses (Fig. 6.3):

- *Relapsing-remitting (RRMS)*: where symptoms may occur and then remit over the course of many years.

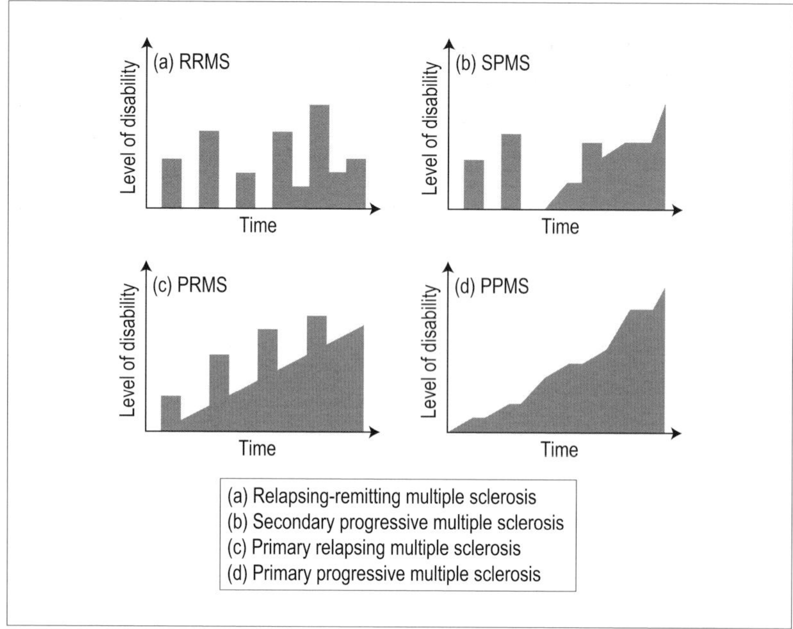

Fig. 6.3 Multiple sclerosis by progression pattern.

- *Secondary progressive (SPMS)*: where symptoms may initially present with a relapsing-remitting course but become gradually more progressive. After a number of years, some sufferers of RRMS may pass into a secondary progressive phase characterized by a gradual deterioration of the condition between relapses.
- *Progressive relapsing (PRMS)*: where symptoms demonstrate a progressive course from onset but with some relapses and recovery.
- *Primary progressive (PPMS)*: where symptoms demonstrate a progression of decline from onset. There is a gradual progression of the condition with no remission.

Variant forms of the condition also exist and include:

- *Benign MS*: this form of MS does not worsen over time and results in no permanent disability. The term is used to describe the condition in patients who have had MS for 10 to 15 years without developing any serious and enduring disability and who initially were categorized as having the RRMS form.
- *Malignant MS (also known as Marburg's variant)*: a very aggressive form of the condition; decline occurs very quickly. It is associated with severe axonal loss and progression is rapid, leading to severe disability in a relatively short period of time. Typically, Marburg's is preceded by a fever and associated with younger patients.
- *Devic's disease (also known as neuromyelitis optica)*: a rare condition of the CNS characterized by bilateral optic neuritis (an inflammation and

demyelination of the optic nerve resulting in a variety of symptoms including blurred vision, reduced visual acuity, changes in colour vision, blindness and pain), followed by inflammation in the spinal cord causing transverse myelopathy associated with both motor and sensory dysfunction in those parts of the limbs and trunk supplied by nerves arising in the spinal cord at or below the point of inflammation.
- *Balo's concentric sclerosis*: another rare condition very similar to MS but demonstrating concentric rings of demyelination in the cerebral white matter on MRI; it is more common in China and the Philippines than elsewhere.

The symptoms of MS vary according to the area of the CNS affected and the severity of involvement. Presentation, therefore, varies from patient to patient as symptoms relapse, remit, or fluctuate along with other physiological changes or with environmental conditions. Box 6.4 provides a non-exhaustive list of many of the symptoms associated with MS. Of course, few of these symptoms are exclusive to MS and can occur with other conditions. However, the breadth of symptomatology shown here underscores the very wide range of potential symptom presentations that can occur.

In the early stages, the most commonly observed symptoms include: motor disturbances such as weakness, stiffness, problems with coordination; visual

Box 6.4 The symptoms of multiple sclerosis

Motor, coordination and balance
Paresis
Hemiparesis
Quadraparesis
Parapelegia
Hemiplegia
Tetraplegia
Quadraplegia
Myoclonus
Spasticity
Intention tremor
Ataxia
Dysphagia
Reduced proprioception
Dysmetria
Dysdiadochokinesia
Vertigo

Sensory
Paraesthesia
Anaethesia
Neuralgia

Visual
Diplopia
Nystagmus
Ophthalmoplegia
Optic neuritis

Neuropsychological
Cognitive dysfunction
Dementia
Emotional dysfunction

Other
Urinary incontinence
Urinary retention
Urinary hesitancy
Constipation
Faecal incontinence
Anorgasmy
Erectile dysfunction
Gastroeosphageal reflux
Epilepsy
Sleep disorder
Fatigue
Uhthoff's sign

disturbances such as blurred vision, double vision, blindness, eye pain; sensory disturbances such as numbness, tingling, or a pins-and-needles sensation. Less commonly observed early symptoms include: balance problems such as dizziness; bladder disturbances such as urinary incontinence or a loss of bladder sensation.

As MS progresses, however, these symptoms may become more significant and include increasing motor deficits, spasticity, tremor, ataxia, sensory difficulties, urinary incontinence and/or urinary retention, constipation, sexual dysfunction in both males and females, and both cognitive and emotional dysfunction.

Epidemiology

Amongst young adults, MS is the most common disease of the CNS. Onset before the age of 15 years is rare, while later onset after the age of 40 years is usually associated with a more rapid progression and greater morbidity (Arnett 2003). According to the Multiple Sclerosis Trust around 85 000 people in the UK suffer with MS, with a sex ratio of females to males of 2:1. Progression of the condition is generally also more rapid in females than males (Kolb & Whishaw 1996).

Environmental factors are suspected in MS development as there appears to be a prevalence rate dependence on latitude. That is to say that the disorder is more prevalent in temperate zones further away from the equator. Again, figures from the Multiple Sclerosis Trust suggest an increased prevalence in Scotland and Canada as opposed to rates in Central America, and equatorial Asia and Africa.

Pathology

The patchy destruction of myelin, the insulation substance sheathing nerve fibres, is the signature marker of MS. When demyelination occurs, there is an accompanying blockage or disruption of nerve impulses and, thus, the processes controlled by the nerve pathways involved become interrupted. The demyelination, for reasons that are yet to be fully understood, spontaneously comes to a halt after an indeterminate period and scarring occurs, forming the characteristic multiple, discrete plaques observed.

Once the inflammation caused by this process terminates, it is possible for damaged myelin to be replaced by the process of remyelination. Naturally, whether this occurs depends on the damage sustained by the surrounding oligodendrocytes. However, generally speaking, nerve axons tend to be preserved since the destruction of the myelin sheath does not necessarily result in the destruction of neuronal tissue. Nevertheless, areas that have been remyelinated tend to possess a thinner layer of myelin than unaffected areas. Such changes tend to reduce the efficiency of the affected nerve tissues and, of course, if several episodes of exacerbation occur in the same area, there is a consequent effect on the degree of remyelination.

After the first appearance of symptoms the course of the condition is unpredictable and extremely variable. Patients may have several relapses during 1 year while others may go for some years without a relapse. A patient experiencing a number of frequent relapse episodes during several years may subsequently enter a phase where no relapses are experienced for a number of years. The symptoms experienced by these patients may be the same during subsequent relapses or they may be different, depending on the region of the CNS involved.

As already stated, the most common sites for MS plaque formation are in the periventricular regions of the brain, the optic nerves, brainstem, cerebellum, and spinal cord. However, the condition can strike at any part of the CNS, both in the white and grey matter, giving rise to the wide range of symptoms observed. For example, because of the greater length of nerve fibres associated with the leg muscles, the myelin sheathing of these axons appear to be particularly exposed and, thus, demonstrate a greater level of involvement (Lezak 1995).

Aetiology

MS is not a fatal condition. Nor is it infectious or contagious. However, the precise mechanism of its development is still unknown. It is thought that the disorder may have components associated with environmental factors, infection, the effects of a virus, or genetics. At present the best explanation for the causation of MS probably lies in a theory of autoimmune response, which suggests that the blood–brain barrier is somehow breached, exposing the proteins of myelin to the body's immune system. These proteins then activate the immune response leading to the breakdown of myelin (Ebers 1986).

As regards the other risk factors that have also been defined, as mentioned previously, geographic latitude appears to be related to development. With the exception of Japan, there appears to be a greater prevalence of MS the further one moves from the equator (Frohman 2003). These observations also indicate that, whatever the environmental factor that is related to MS development, the initial impact occurs during childhood. This is reflected in observations of the condition's frequency in migrant populations, suggesting that those migrating after the age of 15 years will demonstrate the same incidence rates as their country of origin, while those migrating before the age of 15 years will not (Whittaker & Benveniste 1990).

Genetic factors may also play a role in the development of MS (Dyment et al 2004). Although the observed link is tenuous in comparison to other genetic disorders, there is some evidence that suggests that incidence rates are higher amongst children who have a parent suffering from MS, while other work suggests a possible genetic protection from the disorder in different ethnic groups (Cree et al 2004).

Viral infections have also been implicated in MS development. Suggestions range from the triggering of MS through childhood exposure to pathogens to the effects of adult viral acquisition (Levin et al 2005) with viral infection causing an autoimmune response in susceptible individuals.

Of course, no specific aetiology has yet been defined and it is important to remember that the interplay of these various strands of research could, in time, bring about a multifactorial explanation for the causation of MS. For example, a genetically susceptible individual may be exposed to an environmental or viral trigger for the condition, producing the hallmark autoimmune response of demyelination.

Neuropsychological symptoms

Like so many of the disorders of the CNS, the neuropsychological changes associated with MS can produce a wide array of cognitive and emotional dysfunctions, with estimates of cognitive dysfunction ranging from 30 to 70%. Partly, this is due to the nature of the disorder, occurring in apparently random areas of the CNS tissues, and partly because of the variations that occur with time and the severity of an episode of relapse.

The pattern of development of MS plaques within the CNS, then, appears almost at random in the individual patient. The course and expression of the condition is, therefore, unpredictable. The cognitive deficits arising from the formation of these MS plaques will, likewise, be highly individual and unpredictable. Nevertheless, as already observed, MS appears to preferentially affect certain areas of the CNS. There are, therefore, some general commonalities in presentation.

MS, it has also been suggested, meets the criteria for what is described as a subcortical dementia. Briefly, a subcortical dementia is a condition distinct from a cortical dementia such as Alzheimer's disease, primarily affecting subcortical structures; for example Parkinson's disease (see specific section on Parkinson's disease) and Huntington's disease (see specific section on Alzheimer's disease and the other dementias).

These conditions, of course, can occur without cognitive symptoms. However, when these do appear there are some similarities in presentation that have led some to classify them as a category of dementia. These cognitive deficits include a slowing of information processing, poor problem solving, impairments of abstraction, memory deficits, impaired visuospatial abilities, personality changes, and mood disturbances (Cummings & Benson 1984).

Obviously, such a brief definition of subcortical dementia is extremely oversimplified and the reader is directed to the more comprehensive description given by Lezak (1995). It must also be remembered that while a large number of sufferers with MS may present with cognitive difficulties, the great majority of cases demonstrate only a relatively mild deficit, while only a few will qualify for a diagnosis of dementia.

In terms of the cognitive deficits associated with MS it is important to distinguish between primary and secondary causes. Primary factors are those that are the direct result of damage to CNS tissues. Secondary factors are those that occur as a result of the condition; for example fatigue, depression or anxiety. Secondary factors, obviously, will have an effect on neuropsychological performance and, more importantly, represent a reversible element of the condition.

With this caveat in mind, then, perhaps the most frequently observed cluster of problems in MS involves attention and speed of information processing. Many patients demonstrate difficulties with tasks requiring quick and complex information processing that make demands on working memory skills, with the result that patients often have difficulty with following conversations or keeping track of presented information such as in television programmes.

Other common problems in MS that have been reported widely are memory disorders (Litvan et al 1988). Typically, these deficits are observed as difficulties with recall rather than recognition memory, which is very rarely impaired (Rao 1986). The most common problems are with the encoding and/or retrieval of both visual and verbal material and are usually observed as immediate and delayed recall deficits on neuropsychological tests (Arnett 2003). Such deficits generally lead patients, when unprompted, to fail in the recall of information such as appointments or to take care of actions such as remembering to take medications.

Patients with MS also very often manifest problems in visuospatial performance. In practice, however, it is difficult to determine whether these difficulties are simply a manifestation of defects in visual perception, such as blurred vision, or disorders of higher visuospatial functioning. Indeed, it may also be that the other cognitive problems experienced by sufferers may well contribute to the performance impairment observed in these patients (Fennell & Smith 1990).

Executive skills too can be affected by MS. Problems can occur with cognitive flexibility, planning ability, organization, problem solving, reasoning, strategy formation and application, abstraction, concept formation, foresight and judgement. In practice, this is often manifest as problems with thought organization, and difficulties with the planning and organization of everyday actions such as shopping or preparing meals, etc.

With regard to language functioning, problems in the mechanical production of speech, such as hyperphonia, are common. However, disorders of the cognitive skills related to language, such as aphasia, agraphia and alexia, are rare, although some difficulties can be observed in verbal fluency. It is, however, important to distinguish these latter deficits from the more mechanical contributions of motor slowing and other cognitive problems, such as attentional difficulties, speed of information processing or memory impairments.

In terms of the emotional disorders associated with MS, it is not surprising to discover that depression and anxiety occur frequently in MS populations. These emotional disorders are most likely normal reactions to a devastating diagnosis suggesting a lifelong debilitating disease, the experience of fluctuating physical impairment, a reduced quality of life, poor support and uncertainty, etc.

It has also been suggested, however, that the depression accompanying MS, whilst representing a reaction to circumstances, might also be related to organic rather than functional factors. That is to say, the features of depression associated with the condition may also be related to structural changes within the brain. Evidence pointing to this link indicates that patients with MS are more likely to experience depression than normal controls (Fassbender et al 1998) and, indeed, those patients with similarly debilitating neurological conditions (Whitlock & Siskind 1980).

Treatment

Unfortunately, at present there is no cure for MS. However, pharmacological therapies can help to reduce the frequency and severity of relapses. Some medications may even slow the progression of the disorder. In addition, rehabilitation intervention from occupational therapists, speech and language therapists, and neuropsychologists can help in symptom management.

With regard to medication treatments for MS, these fall broadly into three categories: medications that are used to treat relapses episodes; medications used to alter the course of the disorder; and medications used to manage the symptoms of the disorder.

A standard treatment for relapses in MS is corticosteriods, for example methylprednisolone. Such drugs do not affect the long-term course of the disorder or, indeed, the degree of recovery. They do, however, improve the rate of recovery following relapse.

Drugs that act to modify the course of certain forms of the disorder include the beta inteferons, glatiramer acetate, azathioprine, cyclophosphamide methotrexate, and mitoxantrone. These drugs reduce the frequency and severity of relapses by acting either upon the immune system or by working directly with the myelin sheath surrounding nerve tissue.

As a result of their action in reducing relapse frequency and severity, these medications have only been found to be effective in cases of RRMS and in some cases of SPMS. In PPMS, these medications are ineffective. As yet, therefore, no equivalent treatments for PPMS exist.

The medications that are used to manage the various symptoms of MS are manifold and not necessarily specific to the condition. For example, this group of drugs might include benzodiazepines as muscle relaxants, ibuprophen for pain relief, botulinum toxin for spasticity, and amitriptyline for depression. An exhaustive examination of this group, therefore, is beyond the scope of this book.

One exception to this rule, however, is the use of cannabis by many MS sufferers for symptom management and, more recently, research into the clinical utility of prescribing cannabis derivatives. Over the years a great many patients have reported that cannabis is useful in the management of their symptoms. Clinical trials have also produced some evidence of its effectiveness. However, the evidence from such studies remains unclear and research into this area continues.

Summary

MS is an inflammatory condition of the CNS. Inflammation causes damage to the myelin sheath surrounding nerve fibres resulting in a disturbance of normal nerve impulses. The manner in which damage to the nerve's insulating material occurs, results in a number of different courses. The physical and neuropsychological symptoms presented in MS vary in relation to the area of the CNS affected and can also alter with other physiological and environmental conditions. Treatment tends to be symptomatic, although, in certain cases, there are medications that can be used to alter the course of the disorder or improve the rate of recovery from relapse.

PARKINSON'S DISEASE AND PARKINSONISM

Overview

Parkinson's disease primarily affects movement. It is one of a number of progressive neurological disorders and results, principally, from the depletion of the neurotransmitter substance, dopamine. However, the disease can be present for many years before dopamine levels are sufficiently depleted to produce the characteristic motor symptoms of the disorder. Parkinsonism, however, although resembling Parkinson's disease can have a very different aetiology. In this section, then, our aim is to distinguish between these disorders and define the neurological and neuropsychological characteristics of each.

Description

Although similar in presentation, it should be remembered that Parkinson's disease (PD) and parkinsonism are not one and the same. PD, as the term implies, refers to a specific disease, whereas parkinsonism relates to symptoms arising as a manifestation of a variety of other conditions (Tröster 1998). We will look at this distinction in more detail later. First, however, we will consider idiopathic PD, the primary pathological entity.

Initially referred to as the shaking palsy, PD was first described by James Parkinson in 1817. It is a progressive neurodegenerative disease characterized by signs such as tremor, slowness of movement, rigidity and postural abnormalities. The most outstanding features of PD are: a motor disorder associated with an inability to produce movement (akinesia), a slowness of movement (bradykinesia), an involuntary rigid posture, a rigid flexion of the limbs, disorders of equilibrium and posture that result in a flexed trunk position and shuffling gait, and a resting tremor that is interrupted by volitional movement.

The central features of PD stem from disruption of the neural pathways responsible for the control and initiation of movement. Often, these appear unilaterally, affecting only one side of the body, with symptoms eventually becoming bilateral. In some rare cases, PD may be bilateral from the outset.

Generally, the symptoms of PD can be categorized as either positive (those that are not seen in the 'normal' population) or negative (symptoms that represent the absence of a behaviour or inability to engage in an activity). These symptoms include:

- *Resting tremor*: an alternating movement of the limbs when at rest, which is often referred to as 'pill-rolling' tremor because the motion resembles a small object being rolled between the thumb and fingers. There may also be a postural tremor. It should also be noted that the tremor stops when voluntary movement takes place and stops during sleep.

- *Bradykinesia*: a slowness of movement.
- *Hypokinesia*: a reduced amplitude or size of movement.
- *Akinesia*: a poverty or absence of normal unconscious movement, the most frequently seen examples being the loss of natural arm swing when walking, a blankness of facial expression, and reduced blinking. This area of symptomatology also includes 'freezing', an inability to initiate voluntary movement and difficulties in the production of fine movements such as those required to control handwriting, resulting in a condition known as micrographia, a decrease in handwriting size.
- *Kinesia paradoxica*: some patients with PD exhibit a paradoxical sensitivity to externally evoked motor activation, resulting in sudden and usually brief episodes of symptom remission.
- *Muscular rigidity*: an increased muscular rigidity in both flexor and extensor muscles and, therefore, a stiffness of the limbs, demonstrated by resistance to passive movement. Often the limb moves as if one were bending a lead pipe. Movement appears in set degrees and the limb then stays in the flexed position. This is also referred to as 'cogwheel rigidity'.
- *Postural instability*: usually occurring later in the course of the disease, this is characterized by difficulty in maintaining a body part in the normal position relative to other body parts, and a disorder of equilibrium producing difficulties in standing or sitting when unsupported. Often this results in a tendency to stumble and fall.
- *Festination*: linked to both the motor symptoms and postural problems associated with PD, festination (from the Latin festinare, meaning to hasten) refers to a rapid walking style of short, shuffling steps whereby patients initiate walking and then appear to hurry or hasten to catch up with themselves.
- *Disturbances of speech*: consisting mainly of difficulties in the physical production of sound and in changing the tone of the voice.

In addition to the motor dysfunction of PD, some patients may also experience a number of secondary symptoms. These include depression in approximately 40% of cases and dementia in approximately 30% of cases.

Importantly, it should also be noted that the presence of both tremor and rigidity can mask other symptoms which may be a byproduct of PD treatment. To illustrate, dyskinesia, involuntary movements caused by high doses of, or long exposure to, levodopa, can be mistaken for tremor, while dystonia, an impairment of muscle tone and another side-effect of drug treatment, can be confused with rigidity.

As regards the course of the disease, the motor symptoms of PD emerge only after dopamine levels have been significantly reduced. In its early or prodromal stage, dopamine reduction is not at a sufficient level to reveal motor symptoms and this may last for 20 years or more. However, as the disease slowly progresses, the obvious motor symptoms become apparent and a decline over time can be observed. Patients with PD, nevertheless, often survive for 10–15 years after initial diagnosis and comparative rates for mortality in medicated patients tend to be almost that of the unaffected population.

Epidemiology

In the UK, PD affects somewhere between 1 in 500 and 1 in 1000 of the population. The average age of onset is between about 55 and 65 years. This incidence risk increases by approximately 1% in those over the age of 65 years and because of this it is generally associated with the elderly. However, approximately 10% of cases of PD occur in those below the age of 40 years.

In terms of sex differences, some studies have stated that men are three times more likely to be diagnosed with PD than women, while others have claimed a roughly equal incidence between the sexes.

Interestingly, PD occurs worldwide, but the incidence of the disease differs significantly between countries. For example, the prevalence of PD in Africa and China is much lower than elsewhere.

As mentioned earlier, there is a difference between PD and parkinsonism and, indeed, PD forms part of a larger category of parkinsonian disorders characterized by a similar set of symptoms. PD accounts for approximately 80% of these Parkinsonian disorders. Of these, some 95% of cases demonstrate no specific cause and are termed idiopathic. The remaining 5% of cases suggest a genetic link and are described as familial or inherited.

PD, then, is the most commonly observed degenerative disorder of the motor system and, after Alzheimer's disease, is the second most common neurodegenerative disorder encountered.

Pathology

Degeneration involves a region of the brainstem known as the substantia nigra and an increasingly significant reduction in the levels of the neurotransmitter dopamine (Fig. 6.4). Usually, the typical signs of PD appear when dopamine levels drop to between 10 and 20% of normal.

Lewy bodies, on the other hand, are abnormal protein groupings within cells. They can occur throughout the brain. However, their presence in the

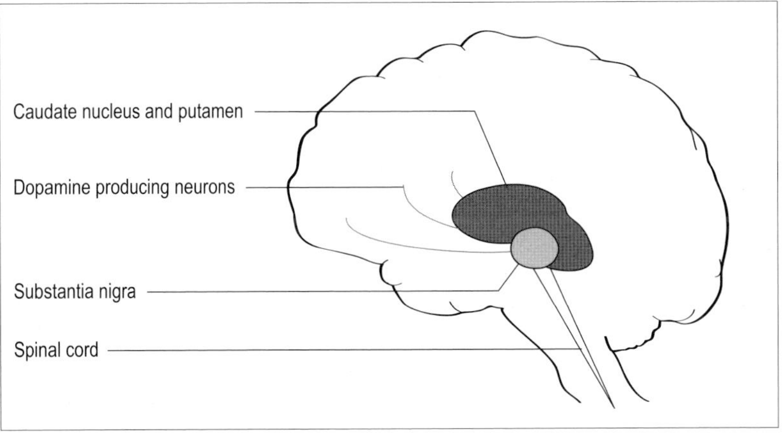

Fig. 6.4 Parkinson's disease.

substantia nigra is associated with PD. The main protein within Lewy bodies is thought to have a function in the uptake of dopamine, but the role of Lewy bodies in PD as a whole is not yet fully understood.

Aetiology

At present it is not possible to suggest a specific cause for PD. A number of risk factors have, however, been defined. First, as stated above, there is an increasing incidence of PD with age, although it must be remembered that PD does form part of the normal aging process. Secondly, and again previously mentioned, certain cases of PD are associated with a genetic link. Therefore, a family history of the disease can also be viewed as a risk factor.

One interesting feature in PD research has, however, come to light. This is the observation that PD appears to occur less frequently in smokers, suggesting that something inhaled from the burning of tobacco could act as some form of reverse risk factor (Baron 1986). This finding, nevertheless, has been disputed with arguments suggesting that, despite the consistency of these findings, smokers tend to be younger and that since PD is generally a late-onset disease, smokers do not tend to survive long enough to develop symptoms (Rajput et al 1987).

Neuropsychological symptoms

A wide range of cognitive impairments can be observed in patients with PD. Many of these deficits are similar to those observed in damage to the frontal lobes and could suggest that changes in the levels of dopamine could have an affect on performance (Gotham et al 1988). On the whole, as with the motor symptoms of PD, medicated patients tend to show a relatively slow decline in cognition, with greater levels of decline tending to be observed in patients with an earlier onset and rigidity and akinesia rather than tremor as their primary symptom.

Bradyphrenia, a slowing of thought processes, often occurs in many PD patients (Cummings 1986). Like the bradykinesis associated with motor functioning, a slowing of mental functions can often be observed. This, in turn, can have an influence on a number of other cognitive skills and, therefore, probably contributes to a poorer performance in other domains. This same slowing of the thought processes is also associated with depression, which we will look at in more detail later.

Attentional problems also tend to be common in PD, with impairments most likely to be observed on more complicated tasks requiring a shifting or maintenance of attention (Cummings 1986). These impairments can, again, affect other cognitive skills such as memory functions.

However, apart from the expected influence of attentional problems, memory difficulties are a common finding in PD (Anderson 1994). This appears to be related to deficits in the ability to organize, search and query memory. Such a pattern of memory deficit tends to suggest the involvement of the frontal lobes.

This suggestion of frontal lobe involvement is reflected in the observation that many PD patients demonstrate neuropsychological symptoms similar to those in cases of lesions to the frontal lobes (Caltagirone et al 1989). Thus, many PD patients also appear to exhibit deficits in maintaining and shifting attention, novel reasoning, initiating behaviour, cognitive flexibility and novel problem-solving. It is useful, however, to be aware that once a PD patient has formulated a solution to a particular problem, they tend to perform at near normal rates (Saint-Cyr & Taylor 1992).

Verbal functions in PD, however, are likely to remain intact, although, as might be expected, there is an overall reduction in output, and hypokinetic dysarthria, a deficit in the mechanical production of speech, is common. Nevertheless, verbal disturbances do occur and these are usually associated with word-finding and poor fluency (Lees & Smith 1983). A disturbance of writing skills, known as micrographia, can also be observed. This tends to parallel the problems observed in speech and results in a small, cramped, and rough mechanical writing style.

Visuospatial deficits are also frequently reported in PD and although right-left orientation appears, for the most part, to remain unimpaired, there appears to be a gradual decline in other areas of visuospatial perception (Levin et al 1991).

The evaluation of cognitive deficits in PD is complicated by the presence of depression, one of the most commonly reported emotional dysfunctions associated with the illness. As mentioned earlier, it is generally accepted that depression appears to occur in approximately 40% of cases (Starkstein et al 1990), although, depending on the source, this figure can be as low as 20% or as high as 90%.

Nevertheless, debate continues as to whether depression in PD represents an emotional reaction to a progressive illness or a symptom caused by changes in the neurochemistry of the brain (Sano et al 1989). Some studies, for example, suggest that depression does not necessarily correlate with the extent of motor impairment, age, or disease duration and that it may, in some cases, even precede the motor signs of PD. In addition, it has been suggested that PD patients with depression also demonstrate a higher incidence of anxiety and panic disorder (Schiffer et al 1988). Obviously, such findings imply that the depression often seen in PD does not simply occur as a reaction to a potentially disabling chronic illness but that it is more likely to be a symptom of PD, at least in some cases.

Whatever the cause, however, depression is consistently observed as being more prevalent in patients with PD (Soukup & Adams 1996) and this is obviously an important factor when assessing cognitive function (Starkstein et al 1992). To illustrate, studies have demonstrated that there is a negative relationship between depression and cognitive functioning (Tröster et al 1995), which is to say that the more severe the depression, the more significant the cognitive deficits observed.

It should also be kept in mind that some of what we observe to be the outward symptoms of depression may also be related to the PD itself. For example, a reduction in facial expression and motor retardation may be evident in both depression and PD. This then requires the observer to establish whether or not the patient does indeed have a depressed mood.

Finally, a prodromal or early personality feature has also been associated with PD by some researchers. This personality profile is characterized by depression, rigidity, introversion, pessimism, seriousness, stoicism and restricted emotional expression (Stacy & Jankovic 1992). Such observations again, however, beg the question of the chicken and the egg. That is to say, do these characteristics emerge as a separate entity, resulting from the early neurochemical changes associated with PD; or do they result from the effect of PD on patients?

It has been suggested that such personality characteristics are a pathological consequence of the neurological changes associated with the disease that may occur many years before there is evidence of motor symptoms (Lohr & Wisniewski 1987). On the other hand, others have suggested that such characteristics may cause individuals to be heavier consumers of water, thus increasing their risk of exposure to possibly toxic substances (Paulson & Dadmehr 1991).

Hallucinations in PD are generally of the visual type and affect approximately 25% of patients. Often these hallucinations are considered to be a side-effect of treatment. However, it appears likely other factors may be involved (Fénelon et al 2000).

Commonly, patients with PD report both minor and more complex forms of visual hallucination. In their minor form, the most frequent is the presence hallucination, where patients report the vivid sensation of the presence of someone either in the room with them or, less often, behind them. Another type of minor presentation is the passage hallucination consisting of brief visions of people or animals passing by the patient. More complex formed visual hallucinations tend to involve people or animals and sometimes other beings such as demons.

The occurrence of hallucinations tends to increase with the duration of the illness and the severity of motor symptoms. In addition, in the case of the more complex hallucinations, there tends to be an increased prevalence with age and the presence of dementia.

Studies of these phenomena, however, suggest that rather than there being a simple medication-linked explanation for their emergence, there is, more likely, a complex interaction between numerous variables (Barnes & David 2001). These probably include cognition, emotion, sensory and perceptual factors, sleep/wake cycles, medication and other environmental factors.

Parkinsonism and Parkinson's plus syndromes

In addition to PD, there are a number of other neurological disorders that can exhibit similar symptoms but that are not considered to be primary idiopathic PD. In these disorders, as with PD, the substantia nigra is damaged, or the activity of its cells is blocked or cells are destroyed. In each case, dopamine levels are reduced and motor symptoms begin to manifest themselves.

These secondary parkinsonisms come in three main forms: acquired, heredodegenerative, and multiple system degenerations (the so called Parkinson's plus syndromes). The overlap between the presentation of these conditions and PD is considerable with investigations conducted at autopsy to confirm the accuracy of clinical diagnosis suggesting that approximately 20% of cases are misdiagnosed (Soukup & Adams 1996). Box 6.5 provides a list of the various classifications of these aetiologies.

Treatment

There is, at present, no cure for the ongoing neurodegeneration that occurs in PD. It is, however, possible to treat the symptoms. The treatment of PD underwent a dramatic change in the 1960s with the introduction of levodopa to enhance dwindling dopamine levels and it remains the most effective pharmacological treatment for PD.

Levodopa increases the levels of dopamine in the brain where the administration of dopamine itself would be ineffective because this sub-

Box 6.5 Parkinsonism and the Parkinson's plus syndromes aetiologies

Acquired parkinsonism

Infectious
CJD, viral encephalitis, syphilis, encephalitis lethargica, HIV, toxoplasmosis

Structural
Hydrocephalus, chronic subdural haematoma, arteriovenous malformation, tumour

Vascular
Mutiple infarcts, basal ganglia infarct

Toxin-induced
Manganese, mercury, carbon monoxide, carbon, cyanide, MPTP (methyl phenyltetrahydropyridine)

Traumatic
Pugilistic encephalopathy

Drug-induced
Dopamine-blocking agents such as antipsychotics, lithium, methyldopa

Heredodegenerative Parkinsonism
Wilson's disease
Huntington's disease
Gaucher's disease
Hallervorden-Spatz disease
Olivopontocerebellar degeneration
Spincocerebellar degeneration

Multiple system degeneration/Parkinson's plus syndromes
Lewy body disease
Shy-Drager syndrome
Progressive supranuclear palsy
Striatonigral degeneration
Parkinson ALS-dementia complex of Guam
Corticobasal ganglionic degeneration

stance will not effectively cross the blood–brain barrier. Being the metabolic precursor of dopamine, however, levodopa will cross this barrier and be converted into dopamine. Today the drug is combined with carbidopa and benserazide to enhance its effects and thus allow for lower doses to be administered.

This lowering of effective doses of levodopa is important because soon after it was introduced it was found that it could, whilst still being effective, produce numerous side-effects. Peak plasma concentration is reached within the first hour after ingestion of the drug. To avoid fluctuations, long-acting preparations such as Sinemet CR have been developed.

Patients generally report a marked response to levodopa at the commencement of therapy. However, these gains are seen to diminish after some years necessitating an increase in dosage. This increases the risk of side-effects which can include mild psychotic symptoms such as paranoid delusions, hallucinations, nightmares, confusion and dyskinesia.

Another complication of levodopa therapy is the 'on-off' phase characterized by time-related dosage intake fluctuations in the motor symptoms of the illness. Usually, these phases appear after a patient has been taking the drug for a number of years and describe the often rapid fluctuations from a state of dysfunctional movement to a state of normal movement and back again. The effect takes its name from patients comparing the experience to an electric switch being turned on or off.

In addition to these dopamine-based therapies, there are also drugs that target the other neurological systems affected by the dopamine decrease. These include the cholinergic and GABAergic (gamma-aminobutyric acid) systems. Normally these systems are inhibited by dopamine and, therefore, become overactive in PD. Anticholinergic substances and GABA antagonists, then, can help to counteract this.

Neurosurgical treatments for PD involve either the lesioning of parts of the brain, the implantation of electrical devices or the implantation of fetal tissues. In approaches that selectively lesion brain regions, the areas responsible for the symptoms are inactivated. These procedures include thalmotomy and pallidotomy and are often used in conjunction with drug therapy.

A similar effect can be achieved by the implantation of a high-frequency stimulator within the tissues of the brain. Such a procedure obviously has the advantage of being reversible, but requires a much higher degree of maintenance and is also more expensive.

The transplantation of fetal nerve cells into the affected area of the brain has demonstrated some promise. However, this work is still experimental and, although these fetal dopamine neuron grafts are able to survive and develop in the adult brain and can deliver long-term relief of symptoms, there is a great deal of work still to be done with regard to cell survival during harvesting and graft survival after implantation.

Finally, while electroconvulsive therapy (ECT) can be used to alleviate the symptoms of depression, it can also be used to improve the rigidity, bradykinesia and tremor associated with PD. For the most part, motor symptom improvement is usually observed before an improvement in mood is seen. However, this improvement is not usually maintained. Nevertheless, the fact that ECT and antidepressant drug therapy can affect both depression and motor symptoms of PD suggests a link between these symptoms.

The challenge for neuropsychology in these cases, then, is the assessment, stabilization and management of presenting neuropsychological symptoms and the support of both the patient and family. This may be achieved through education, the provision of information and advice, and understanding of the neurophysiological processes underlying PD and the addressing of specific problems; for example, the use of external stimuli to overcome 'freezing', and intervention aimed at the emotional problems that can occur as a primary factor or a secondary reaction to the illness and the decompensation that these can produce.

Summary

PD is a progressive neurodegenerative disease characterized by a motor disorder producing akinesia, bradykinesia and tremor. There are also postural difficulties, limb flexion and difficulties with equilibrium. These symptoms result from a progressive reduction in the levels of dopamine within the brain. As yet the cause of PD is unknown. Neuropsychological symptoms vary but can reflect progressive difficulties with frontal lobe functions, the presence of bradyphrenia, attentional difficulties and memory problems. Emotional difficulties with depression and anxiety are also common features. Treatment is primarily through levodopa-based medication, although with increasing dosage there can be unpleasant side-effects.

Parkinsonism and the Parkinson's plus syndromes, on the other hand, like PD result from the damage of dopaminergic cells within the brain. However, these disorders are considered secondary to other causative factors, and while the similarities between these parkinsonism producing disorders and PD is considerable, they are not considered to be primary idiopathic PD.

TRAUMATIC BRAIN INJURY

Overview

Traumatic brain injury represents, perhaps, the single largest source of brain damage in the young. It occurs as a result of mechanical trauma to the skull and underlying tissues and, as a result, either directly or indirectly, can cause the involvement of almost any brain structure. In these circumstances, it is not surprising that a very wide variety of neurological and neuropsychological symptoms can arise from these cases. Here, then, we will attempt to categorize the various different types of trauma, examine some of the primary and secondary effects of injury, and look at some of the neuropsychological impairments that can occur as a result of such trauma.

Description

Synonymous with head injury, traumatic brain injury (TBI) is, by far, the most common cause of brain damage in those under the age of 40 years. TBI constitutes the abrupt physical damage to the brain caused by the head trauma of impacts, such as those produced by road traffic accidents (RTAs) or by the passage of objects through the skull and brain, such as missile wounds. Thus, the major causes of TBIs are motor vehicle accidents, falls, sports injuries, and violent crimes.

More specifically, the Medical Disability Society Working Party Report on the Management of Traumatic Brain Injury (1988) defines TBI as brain injury caused by trauma to the head (including the effects upon the brain of other possible complications of injury, notably hypoxaemia and hypotension, and intracerebral haematoma).

That is to say, that at least in this context, the cause of brain injury comes initially from the influence of an outside force, but includes the secondary complications which can follow such an injury. This includes a lack of oxygen, rising pressure, and swelling in the brain. A TBI, then, can be viewed as a series of events commencing with the initial injury followed by secondary effects.

Thus, primary damage occurs at the time of the injury, caused by mechanical forces of deceleration acting on the brain at impact. This includes direct, focal damage to the brain, or more diffuse injuries such as the disruption of neurons and small blood vessels, while secondary damage can occur minutes, hours, or even days after the initial event and includes injuries caused by intracranial haematoma, intracranial infection, systemic hypoxia, and hypertension/hypotension.

TBIs may also be classified by type and severity. As regards the type of injury sustained, there are three categories: closed, open and crush injuries. Closed head injuries are the most common and are so called because no wound to the scalp or skull is visible; for example when travelling in a motor vehicle that decelerates rapidly on impact with a stationary object. Open or penetrating injuries occur when the skull is penetrated or opened; for example by the passage of a bullet. Finally, crush injuries occur when the head is compressed between two or more other objects; for example when the head is injured by being caught between the wheel of a motor vehicle and the surface of the road.

Alternatively, TBIs may also be categorized by their severity as mild, moderate or severe. The most common of these is the mild or minor head injury, accounting for an estimated 95% of all head injuries (McMillan & Greenwood 1997). Minor head injuries consist of actions such as hitting the head while getting out of a motor vehicle or striking the head against a low shelf. Such injuries may or may not be associated with a brief period of unconsciousness and symptoms can include nausea, headaches, dizziness, reduced concentration, mild memory problems, fatigue and increased sensitivity to light and sound.

Patients with more significant minor head injuries typically have concussion, with concussion defined as physiological injury to the brain without any evidence of structural alteration. If symptoms such as those listed above persist, as is observed in approximately 5% of cases (McMillan & Greenwood 1997), they are referred to as post-concussion syndrome (PCS) which can additionally present with diplopia, blurred vision, emotional lability, sleep disturbances, and both anxiety and depression. Typically, these symptoms are short lived and self-resolving but can persist in some patients for up to a year (Selby 2000).

Moderate head injury may be defined as that which results in a loss of consciousness lasting for between 15 minutes and 6 hours, and a period of post-traumatic amnesia (PTA) of between 6 and 24 hours.

Level of consciousness is typically measured by way of the Glasgow Coma Scale (GCS), the most common method of severity indexing (Teasdale & Jennet 1974). PTA, on the other hand, is the disruption of continuous memory that can accompany head trauma. Memory, in this case, is not represented by the first remembered event following the trauma, as this may simply be an 'island' of recall; instead, PTA refers to the period of time during which the ability to acquire and retain new information is interrupted. PTA, therefore, is a disturbance of the mechanism responsible for ongoing encoding and storage of memory and is, typically, a more accurate predictor of the recovery of function after TBI (Lucas 1998).

Severe head injuries are defined as causing unconsciousness for a period of more than 6 hours but less than 48 hours, with a PTA of more than 24 hours but less than 7 days. Very severe injuries, meanwhile, are associated with unconsciousness of more than 48 hours and a PTA in excess of 7 days.

Epidemiology

Head injury is rated among the five most prevalent neurological conditions affecting the CNS along with cerebrovascular disease, epilepsy, Parkinson's disease and migraine (McMillan & Greenwood 1997). Indeed, according to Headway, the UK's brain injury charity, it is estimated that approximately 1 million people attend hospital each year as a result of head injury.

In terms of the distribution of these cases, the great majority, some 84%, are classified as minor, while 11% and 5% are classified as moderate or severe, respectively (Miller & Jones 1985). That is to say, approximately 250 to 300 cases per 100 000 of the population present with minor head injury, 18 cases per 100 000 of the population with moderate head injury and 8 cases per 100 000 of the population with severe injury (Medical Disability Society 1988).

Sex distribution figures also demonstrate a difference, with consistently higher rates of incidence among males than females (Tennant 1995). In general, males are between two and three times more likely to suffer a head injury than females, while the injuries suffered by males tend to be more severe (Dikmen et al 1995).

Age, however, is also an important factor, with younger age groups tending to be over-represented (McMillan & Greenwood 1997). The greatest vulnerability observed is in those aged between 15 and 29 years, while the ratio of male to female cases demonstrates that males in this age grouping are five times more likely to sustain injuries than females.

One family in every 300 is thought to have a family member with persisting disability caused by head injury, with some 1500 persons per 100 000 of the population severely or profoundly disabled every year (King & Tyerman 2003).

Pathology

TBIs, as mentioned previously, can be closed, penetrating or crush injuries with primary or secondary effects. Primary, direct mechanical trauma is caused as the brain moves backward and forward within the rigid, inelastic skull, as an object passes through the brain tissue, or by way of compression of the brain tissues.

Energy transferred to the skull when the head impacts with an object is dissipated within the head. This energy can be transferred directly to the brain tissues when the brain strikes the interior surface of the skull or by producing an oscillation of the brain within the skull. When the surface of the brain impacts against the skull's interior, this can produce focal cortical contusion or lacerations while rotational movements of the brain within the skull can cause white matter pathways to strain and tear, blood vessels to haemorrhage, and other support structures to be damaged.

Coup type contusions arise at the point of impact when the brain is accelerated within the skull. These contusions may also be associated with scalp or skull injuries but this is not always the case. Contre-coup type contusions arise opposite the point of impact and are caused by abrupt deceleration of the brain within the skull. Often these are more severe contusions occurring as the brain moves rapidly over the irregularities of the skull's interior and especially over the internal surfaces of the frontal and temporal areas which are particularly coarse and uneven.

Frequently more damaging, however, are the physical rotational and acceleration/deceleration forces present at the time of the impact. Such forces can produce the rupture of blood vessels and a shearing of tissues giving rise to diffuse axonal injuries. Diffuse axonal injuries are a pulling apart of the axons and disruption of the cell bodies occurring as a consequence of the momentary distortion of the brain's shape and density at the time of impact (Williamson et al 1996).

In penetrating head injuries, damage arises from the destruction of brain tissue by the impinging object. However, the amount of damage done to the tissues is related to the energy translated to the brain by the damaging event (Grafman & Salazar 1987). In the case of the missile wounds produced by bullets, for example, air compressed in front of the bullet causes an explosive effect on entering the skull. If the bullet is of the low velocity kind, damage is typically restricted to the missile's track. At higher velocities, however, damage tends to extend beyond the missile track (Lucas 1998).

In addition to these primary factors, a host of secondary injuries can also occur as a result of the nature and extent of direct mechanical trauma. These include haemorrhage and the formation of intracerebral haematomas, cerebral ischaemia, hypotension, cerebral oedema and infection.

The stress forces present at the time of impact can produce a tearing of blood vessels with the resultant haematoma acting as a space-occupying lesion. Intracerebral haematomas can be either large or small. Larger formations, however, tend to be associated with higher rates of morbidity because of their proximity to the brainstem.

Subdural haematomas generally result from a rupture of the bridging veins that follow the surface of the brain. Such haematomas, therefore, tend to form at lower venous pressure and may develop over time. Extradural haematomas, meanwhile, result from injuries to the extradural arteries and tend to follow the course of skull fractures. These haematomas can be quite large and often follow skull fractures over these arteries. They can also result in significant complications as they compress the surrounding cerebral tissue.

Cerebral ischaemia commonly occurs after severe head injury and can be caused by the hypoxia/anoxia of haemorrhage, cardiopulmonary failure, or the compression effects of increased intracranial pressure. It may also occur as a result of reduced cerebral perfusion secondary to hypotension.

Cerebral oedema is also a common complication of TBI. It may develop over minutes or hours following injury and can occur with or without the formation of intracranial haematoma. Frequently, in more severe cases, such oedemas can prove fatal and emergency neurosurgical intervention may be required to reduce intracranial pressure.

Infection, although it may also feature as a secondary source of injuries in closed head injury, is more common in penetrating head injuries because of their invasive nature. Therefore, both early meningitis and later brain abscesses can both be observed in this form of injury.

Finally, a rare but potentially life-threatening and, therefore, important condition to remember in TBI pathology is second impact syndrome. This is caused by repeated concussion over a short period of time. Typically, this condition can be seen in contact sports such as boxing and arises when an individual receives a second trauma whilst not yet fully recovered from the first. In such cases, even a minor second injury can produce significant effects because of a disturbance of the auto-regulation of cerebral blood flow, which increases cerebral blood volume. This, in turn, increases intracranial pressure, reduces cerebral perfusion and increases the risk of cerebral herniation (Lucas 1998). Obviously, those who have suffered more significant injuries are more at risk for this condition. This is because they have already suffered a TBI and may be at even greater risk for sustaining further injury because of the neurological and neuropsychological consequences of the initial trauma.

Aetiology

Whilst there are many mechanisms involved in the causation of TBI, and incidence rates may vary in response to other factors such as age, sex, and geography, etc., there are still a number of commonalities in general aetiology.

By far the most common cause of TBI remains RTAs, accounting for some 45% of all injuries. This category includes events such as collisions between motor vehicles, impacts between pedestrians and motor vehicles, and bicycle accidents (which account for approximately 20% of the head injuries observed in children).

The next most common causes of TBIs are: falls, accounting for approximately 30% of injuries; occupational accidents, accounting for approximately 10% of injuries; sports and recreational accidents, accounting for approximately 10% of injuries; and assaults accounting for approximately 5% of injuries.

Neuropsychological symptoms

In the case of mild closed head injuries, patients commonly report difficulties with speed of information processing, poor attentional skills and disturbed memory. Typically, there are difficulties noted with increased distractibility, reduced concentration, mild deficits in verbal and visual short-term memory, and problems with word retrieval. Emotionally, there may also be increased irritability, frustration, depression and anxiety, and loss of confidence secondary to these cognitive impairments.

Often these complaints correlate with the severity of PCS reported and, in the majority of cases, impairments are not expected to last more than 1 month (Levin et al 1987). There are patients, however, whose symptoms persist for longer periods (Leininger et al 1990) and they frequently demonstrate a greater degree of emotional disturbance, suggesting the possibility that feelings of depression or anxiety, etc. might represent a reaction to the cognitive inefficiency suffered rather than simply being a manifestation of cerebral damage.

Moderate injuries can and do produce a wider variety of neuropsychological symptoms than do mild injuries. Again, the most common complaints are headaches, reduced speed of information processing, attentional problems and memory difficulties, with patients continuing to demonstrate significant difficulties 3 months post trauma (Rimel et al 1982). In many cases, frontal lobe involvement may be suspected with behavioural or personality change and difficulties with the executive functions of planning and self-monitoring. PCS is often present and such may be the magnitude of the psychoemotional trauma that post traumatic stress (PTS) is evident. For example, there might be difficulties associated with the phobic avoidance of situations similar to those at the time when the injury took place; for instance there may be significant anxiety generated by being a passenger in a motor vehicle.

Severe injuries, however, because of their very nature, present us with a wide variety of both neurological and neuropsychological impairments. For most, there are many physical deficits and disabilities to overcome and for the majority, these will take precedence over cognitive symptoms during the first few months post injury. In the long term, however, these neuropsychological impairments may ultimately prove to have a greater impact on functioning than residual physical disability. Generally speaking, the neuropsychological impairments arising from severe injuries can be grouped into cognitive, behavioural and emotional problems.

Although care must be taken to both appreciate the individual and unique characteristics of each injury and exclude the impact of residual physical disability on performance (e.g. residual dyspraxia will affect performance on neuropsychological tests sensitive to motor impairments), the distribution of cognitive deficits observed here tends to reflect the vulnerability of the frontal and temporal areas to damage and the influence of diffuse axonal injury. Patients with this type of TBI, therefore, while capable of demonstrating dysfunction in almost all areas of cognition, tend to present with problems related to difficulties with speed of information processing, attentional disorders, memory dysfunctions, and executive dysfunctions.

Disturbances of attention and concentration and speed of information processing are common, particularly in those that have experienced injury secondary to rapid deceleration forces, such as those observed in many RTAs. If severe, these attentional problems can be a significant barrier to both assessment and treatment as the sufferer is unable to maintain focus on the task in hand.

Memory disturbances are also common after severe TBI. They tend to present as impairments in long-term and short-term stores, visual and verbal stores, and as problems with the acquisition and retrieval of information. In very significant cases this can produce problems whereby the patient is only aware of immediate events or items and is unable to recall information after the passage of a relatively short period of time. Nevertheless, remote memory and implicit memory generally appear to be spared.

Executive dysfunctions are, again, frequently observed in severe cases. Often these are evidenced as reduced cognitive flexibility, perseveration, difficulties with abstract reasoning, problems with planning and problem-solving, poor initiation, poor adaptation to new or novel situations, lack of insight and diminished awareness, poor social integration, and a reduced awareness of deficit.

A wide range of emotional and neurobehavioural disorders can also be observed in cases of severe TBI. As might be expected, anxiety, depression, anger, frustration and distress feature prominently as reactions to the trauma, as well as the presence of residual disabilities and the adjustments the patient must make. These, by and large, are normal reactions but may be complicated by one or more of the cognitive deficits listed above and may be particularly vulnerable to difficulties with executive functioning.

Difficulties associated with behavioural changes secondary to the trauma, such as disinhibition, impulsivity, increased irritability, aggression, rapid mood swings, emotional lability and personality change may also be present. In part these difficulties may be due to the primary tissue damage of the trauma or its secondary effects.

It must be remembered, however, that the interaction of residual cognitive and physical deficits with the individual patient's psychological and psychoemotional make-up will also play an integral role in the manifestation of these features. For example, patients displaying anger, frustration and irritability may be possessed of emotional dysfunctions related to the trauma. However, they may also be reacting to the cognitive and physical symptoms that same trauma has produced.

Treatment

In the great majority of minor or moderate injuries, no pathophysiological changes are observed and many patients suffer few or no residual symptoms.

In those that do, the neuropsychological focus of treatment is usually on the provision of information, education, reassurance, advice and support with, if necessary, regular monitoring. The aim, therefore, is both to assess the severity of any persistent symptoms and the extent to which PCS and/or PTS may be present, and also to offer interventions aimed at educating and normalizing the patient's response to the trauma. It is prudent, however, to be aware that even seemingly minor injuries can produce quite significant impairments in some patients and that repeated minor concussions can have a cumulative effect (Gronwall & Wrightson 1975).

In more severe injuries, however, damage to the brain is typically widespread and improvement in the sufferer's condition typically takes months or even years. During the acute stages, medical management might include the monitoring of elevated ICP, the treatment of hydrocephalus caused by intraventricular haemorrhage, surgical intervention for extradural and subdural haematomas, and the elevation and repair of depressed skull fractures.

As time progresses, however, impairments beyond those of the acute medical management phase become apparent. Generally, the characteristics of these more severe injuries tend to be: seizures; disorders of movement, sensation, speech, swallowing, and continence; problems with attention, memory, language, perception, and executive functions; and emotional disturbances such as depression, anxiety, apathy, agitation, disinhibition and emotional lability.

At this stage, the input of a specialized, multidisciplinary team is warranted in order to deal with the multifaceted nature of these residual deficits in order to minimize disability and maximize independence. Ideally, such a team comprises physicians, nurses, speech and language therapists, physiotherapists, occupational therapists and neuropsychologists. Early in the rehabilitation process, the focus is on the reduction of disabling residual symptomatology. Later, as the patient is judged to be more able to cope both physically and psychologically, the focus is on the matching of skills to anticipated needs upon discharge. Finally, as the patient moves towards community integration, the focus moves towards adjustment and the consolidation of gains made in treatment and the setting and achievement of new goals.

From a neuropsychological perspective, it is generally accepted that, after a more serious TBI, recovery will continue for some 2 to 3 years. However, it is also true to say that that the greater part of neuropsychological improvement takes place within the first 6 to 9 months post injury. Neuropsychological rehabilitation, therefore, should optimally account for this window of opportunity and take full advantage of the acute and post-acute phases to deliver services.

Neuropsychological treatment, in this context, is relatively complex as it addresses not only the engagement of the patient and family with both neuropsychology and other rehabilitation services but also the amelioration and management of presenting neuropsychological impairments.

Again, an aim of assessment and treatment is the evaluation of residual symptoms and the provision of information, education, reassurance, advice and support to both the patient and family. In addition, however, the neuropsychologist's role encompasses the setting of realistic rehabilitation goals, monitoring, the minimization of effects of psychological and emotional processes that can have an additional impact on residual symptoms and, importantly, cognitive rehabilitation, which seeks to maximize function through the restoration or compensation of cognitive deficits.

SUMMARY

TBI represents physical damage to the brain caused by head impacts through: RTAs, falls, sports injuries, and violent crimes; the trauma of projectiles injuries; and the influence of secondary complications following such an injury. They can be classified by type such as: closed, penetrating or crush type injuries, and as minor, moderate or severe injuries. Neuropsychological symptoms vary with the site and severity of the initial injury as well as with the influence of secondary factors and can be complicated by the presence of further emotional difficulties resulting either as a reaction to injury or as a symptom of direct trauma.

CONCLUSION

This chapter has focused on dementia, epilepsy, CVA, MS, TBI and PD, the more common disorders encountered by neuropsychologists, and has examined the accompanying aetiology, pathophysiology, symptoms and neuropsychological profile of each. Sometimes the neuropsychological sequelae of these maladies have occurred in isolation, and sometimes the cognitive and emotional presentations have overlapped to form an often bewildering array of signs and symptoms.

Such a representation of different conditions serves to underscore both the folly of attempting to localize too closely explicit cognitive functions with specific structures within the brain, as well as highlighting the complexity of neurocognitive skills and the fabric of tissues that underpins them.

Dementia is defined as a global, progressive, and typically irreversible decline in higher mental functioning beyond that which might be expected to occur in normal aging. Divided into primary and secondary dementias, there is, at present, no treatment for primary dementias that can arrest or reverse the progressive degeneration associated with these conditions.

CVAs, meanwhile, are characterized by the sudden onset of focal neurological symptoms. They arise as a result of the interruption or disturbance of the brain's vascular supply, and occur as a consequence of haemorrhage or ischaemia.

Epilepsy, on the other hand, produces seizures resulting from abnormal electrical discharges in the brain. This gives rise to changes in behaviour and levels of consciousness. The term epilepsy is usually associated with recurrent convulsive episodes but the variety of presentation is extremely varied and causes complex motor disturbances, perceptual symptoms, sensory experiences, mood changes, and behavioural and cognitive disturbances.

MS represents an inflammatory condition of the CNS resulting in demyelination of the insulating covering of nerve fibres. The disorder is extremely variable and presents differently in different individuals, following usually four courses: RRMS (where there is relapse and remission over a number of years); SPMS (involving a gradual progression of symptomatology after an initial RRMS period); PRMS (where symptoms are progressive from the onset but with some relapses and recovery); and PPMS (involving a gradual progression of the symptoms with no remission).

Like the dementing processes, PD is a progressive neurodegenerative disease characterized by distinct motor symptoms. It also produces a group of more subtle neuropsychological signs and symptoms and is caused by a reduction in the levels of the neurotransmitter dopamine within the brain.

Finally, TBI represents the most common cause of brain damage in those under the age of 40 years and results from physical damage to the brain caused by the trauma of impacts, or by the passage of objects through the skull and brain. This results in both primary and secondary injury from either external mechanical forces or resultant processes such as oedema, hypoxia or reduced cerebral perfusion, etc. TBIs are classified by type (closed, open or crush injuries) and severity (mild/minor, moderate, or severe).

REFERENCES

Adams R D, Victor M 1993 Epilepsy and other seizure disorders. In: Adams R D, Victor M (eds) Principles of neurology, 5th edn. McGraw-Hill, New York

Aisen P S, Davis K L 1994 Inflammatory mechanisms in Alzheimer's disease: implications for therapy. American Journal of Psychiatry 151:1105–1113

Amieva H, Jacqmin-Gadda H, Orgogozo J et al 2005 The 9 year cognitive decline before dementia of the Alzheimer type: a prospective population-based study. Brain 128:1093–1101

Anderson R M 1994 Practitioner's guide to clinical neuropsychology. Plenum Press, New York

Arnett P A 2003 Neuropsychological presentation and treatment of demyelinating disorders. In: Halligan P W, Kischka U, Marshall J C (eds) Handbook of clinical neuropsychology. Oxford University Press, Oxford

Ballinger A, Patchett S 2004 Saunders' pocket essentials of clinical medicine, 3rd edn. W B Saunders, Edinburgh

Banich M T 1997 Neuropsychology: the neural basis of mental functions. Houghton Mifflin, New York

Barnes J, David A S 2001 Visual hallucinations in Parkinson's disease: a review and phenomenological survey. Journal of Neurology, Neurosurgery and Psychiatry 70:727–733

Baron J A 1986 Cigarette smoking and Parkinson's disease. Neurology 36:1490–1496

Bear D, Levin K, Blumer D et al 1982 Interictal behaviour in hospitalised temporal lobe epileptics: relationship to psychiatric syndromes. Journal of Neurology, Neurosurgery and Psychiatry 45:481–488

Berent S, Giordani B, Lehtinen S et al 1988 Positron emission tomographic scan investigations of Huntington's disease: cerebral metabolic correlates of cognitive function. Annals of Neurology 23:541–546

Blumer D, Benson D F 1975 Personality changes with frontal and temporal lobe lesions. In: Benson D F, Blumer D (eds) Psychiatric aspects of neurologic disease. Grune and Straton, New York

Caltagirone C, Carlesimo A, Nocentini U et al 1989 Defective concept formation in parkinsonians is independent from mental deterioration. Journal of Neurology, Neurosurgery and Psychiatry 52:334–337

Commission on Classification and Terminology of the International League Against Epilepsy 1981 Proposal for revised clinical and electrographic classification of epileptic seizures. Epilepsia 22:493–495

Cree B, Bourdette D, Goodin D et al 2004 Clinical characteristics of African Americans vs Caucasian Americans with multiple sclerosis. Neurology 63:2039–2045

Cull C, Goldstein L H 1997 An introduction to epilepsy. In: Cull C, Goldstein L H (eds) The clinical psychologist's handbook of epilepsy: assessment and management. Routledge, London

Cummings J L 1986 Subcortical dementia: neuropsychology, neuropsychiatry and pathophysiology. British Journal of Psychiatry 149:682–697

Cummings J L, Benson D F 1984 Subcortical dementia: review of an emerging concept. Archives of Neurology 41:874–879

Dikmen S S, Machamer J E, Winn H R et al 1995 Neuropsychological outcome at 1-year post head injury. Neuropsychology 9:80–90

Dyment D A, Ebers G C, Sadovnick A D 2004 Genetics of multiple sclerosis. The Lancet Neurology 3:104–110

Ebers G C 1986 Multiple sclerosis and other demyelinating diseases. In: Asbury A K, McKhann G M, McDonald W I (eds) Diseases of the nervous system: Clinical neurobiology II. W B Saunders, Philadelphia

Engel J 1989 Seizures and epilepsy. F A Davis, Philadelphia

Fassbender K, Schmidt R, Mössner R et al 1998 Mood disorders and dysfunction of the hypothalamic-pituitary-adrenal axis in multiple sclerosis. Archives of Neurology 55:66–72

Fénelon G, Mahieux F, Huon R et al 2000 Hallucinations in Parkinson's disease: prevalence, phenomenology and risk factors. Brain 123(4):733–745

Fennell E B, Smith M C 1990 Neuropsychological assessment. In: Rao S M (ed) Neurobehavioural aspects of multiple sclerosis. Oxford University Press, New York

Fox N C, Warrington E K, Seiffer A L et al 1998 Presymptomatic cognitive deficits in individuals at risk of familial Alzheimer's disease: a longitudinal perspective study. Brain 131:1631–1639

Frohman E M 2003 Multiple sclerosis. Medical Clinics of North America 87:867–897

Galvez S, Masters C, Gajdusek C 1980 Descriptive epidemiology of Creuzfeldt-Jakob disease in Chile. Archives of Neurology 46:935–939

Gibbs C J, Asher D M, Kobrine A et al 1994 Transmission of Creutzfeldt-Jakob disease to a chimpanzee by electrodes contaminated during neurosurgery. Journal of Neurology, Neurosurgery and Psychiatry 57:757–758

Gotham A M, Brown R G, Marsden C D 1988 Frontal cognitive function in patients with Parkinson's disease 'On' and 'Off' Levodopa. Brain 111(2):299–321

Grafman J, Salazar S 1987 Methodological considerations relevant to the comparison of recovery from penetrating and closed head injuries. In: Levin H S, Grafman J, Eisenberg H S (eds) Neurobehavioral recovery from head injury. Oxford University Press, New York

Gray J M, Young A W, Barker W A et al 1997 Impaired recognition of disgust in Huntington's disease gene carriers. Brain 120:2029–2038

Gronwall D, Wrightson P 1975 Cumulative effects of concussion. The Lancet 2:995–997

Hachinsky V, Norris J W 1985 The acute stroke. F A Davis, Philadelphia

Hansen L, Salmon D P, Galasko D 1990 The Lewy body variant of Alzheimer's disease: a clinical and pathological entity. Neurology 40:1–8

Hauser W A, Annegers J F 1993 Epidemiology of epilepsy. In: Laidlaw J, Richens A, Chadwick D (eds) A textbook of epilepsy. Churchill Livingstone, Edinburgh

Herbert D E, Scherr P A, Beckett L A et al 1992 Relation of smoking and alcohol consumption to incident Alzheimer's disease. American Journal of Epidemiology 135:347–355

Heston L L, Mastri A R, Anderson E et al 1981 Dementia of the Alzheimer type. Archive of General Psychiatry 38:1085–1090
Hirose S, Iwata H, Akiyoshi H et al 1999 A novel mutation of CHRNA4 responsible for autosomal dominant nocturnal frontal lobe epilepsy. Neurology 53:1749–1753
Jarvik L F 1988 Aging of the brain: how can we prevent it? The Gerontologist 28:739–747
Kaneko S, Okada M, Iwasa H et al 2002 Genetics of epilepsy: current status and perspectives. Journal of Neuroscience Research 44:11–30
King N S, Tyerman A 2003 Neuropsychological presentation and treatment of head injury and traumatic brain damage. In: Halligan P W, Kischka U, Marshall J C (eds) Handbook of clinical neuropsychology. Oxford University Press, Oxford
Kitamoto T, Tateishi J, Tashima T et al 1986 Amyloid plaques in Creutzfeldt-Jakob disease stain with prion protein antibodies. Annals of Neurology 20:204–208
Kolb B, Whishaw I Q 1996 Fundamentals of human neuropsychology, 4th edn. W H Freeman, New York
Kumar P, Clark M 2005 Clinical Medicine, 6th edn. Elsevier Saunders, Edinburgh
Kurtzke J F 1983 Epidemiology and risk factors in thrombotic brain infarction. In: Harrison M J G, Dyken M L (eds) Cerebral vascular disease. Butterworths, London
Lechtenberg R 1990 Seizure recognition and treatment. Churchill Livingstone, New York
Lees A J, Smith E 1983 Cognitive deficits in the early stages of Parkinson's disease. Brain 106:257–270
Leininger B E, Gramling S E, Farrell A D et al 1990 Neuropsychological deficits in symptomatic minor head injury patients after concussion and mild concussion. Journal of Neurology, Neurosurgery and Psychiatry 53:293–296
Levin B E, Llabre M M, Reisman S et al 1991 Visuospatial impairment in Parkinson's disease. Neurology 41:365–369
Levin H S, Amparo E, Eisenberg H et al 1987 Magnetic resonance imaging and computerized tomography in relation to the neurobehavioral sequelae of mild and moderate head injuries. Journal of Neurosurgery 66:706–713
Levin L I, Munger K L, Rubertone M V et al 2005 Temporal relationship between elevation of Epstein-Barr virus antibody titers and initial onset of neurological symptoms in multiple sclerosis. Journal of the American Medical Association 20:2496–2500
Lezak M D 1995 Neuropsychological assessment, 3rd edn. Oxford University Press, Oxford
Lindsay K W, Bone I, Callander R 1997 Neurology and neurosurgery illustrated, 3rd edn. Churchill Livingstone, Edinburgh
Lishman W A 1987 Organic psychiatry, 2nd edn. Blackwell Scientific, Oxford
Litvan I, Grafman J, Vendrell P et al 1988 Multiple memory deficits in patients with multiple sclerosis. Archives of Neurology 45:607–611
Lohr J B, Wisniewski A A 1987 Movement disorders. Guilford Press, New York
Lovenstone S, Ritchie K 2002 The dementias. The Lancet 360:1759–1766
Lucas J A 1998 Traumatic brain injury and postconcussive syndrome. In: Snyder P, Nussbaum P (eds) Clinical neuropsychology: a pocket handbook for assessment. American Psychological Association, Washington DC
McMillan T, Greenwood R 1997 Head injury. In: Greenwood R, Barnes M, McMillan T et al (eds) Neurological rehabilitation. Psychology Press, Hove
Medical Disability Society 1988 Report of a working party on the management of traumatic brain injury. The Development Trust for the Young and Disabled, London
Mega M S, Cummings J L, Fiorello T et al 1996 The spectrum of behavioural changes in Alzheimer's disease. Neurology 46:130–135
Miller J D, Jones P A 1985 The work of a regional head injury service. The Lancet 1:1141–1144
Moore D P 2001 Textbook of clinical neuropsychiatry. Arnold, London
Navia B A, Cho E, Petito C K et al 1986 The AIDS dementia complex: II Neuropathology. Annals of Neurology 19:525–535
Neary D, Snowden J 1996 Fronto-temporal dementia: nosology, neuropsychology, and neuropathology. Brain and Cognition 31:176–187

Owen F, Poulter M, Lofthouse R et al 1989 Insertion in prion protein gene in familial Creutzfeldt-Jakob disease. The Lancet 1:51–52
Palmini A L, Gloor P, Jones-Gotman M 1992 Pure amnestic seizures in temporal lobe epilepsy. Brain 115:749–769
Paulson G W, Dadmehr N 1991 Is there a premorbid personality typical for Parkinson's disease? Neurology 41(suppl 2):73–76
Perry R H, Irving D, Blessed G et al 1990 Senile dementia of Lewy body type: a clinically and neuropathologically distinct form of Lewy body dementia in the elderly. Journal of Neurological Science 95:119–139
Petry S, Cummings J L, Hill M A et al 1988 Personality alterations in dementia of the Alzheimer type. Archives of Neurology 45:1187–1190
Pincus J H, Tucker G J 1985 Behavioural neurology, 3rd edn. Oxford University Press, Oxford
Poza J J, Saenza A, Martinez-Gil A et al 1999 Autosomal dominant lateral temporal lobe epilepsy: clinical and genetic study of a large Basque pedigree linked to chromosome 10q. Annals of Neurology 45:182–188
Rajput A H, Offord K P, Beard C M et al 1987 A case-control study of smoking habits, dementia and other illnesses in idiopathic Parkinson's disease. Neurology 37:226–231
Rankin E J, Adams R L, Jones H E 1996 Epilepsy and nonepileptic attack disorder. In: Adams R L, Parsons O A, Culbertson J L et al (eds) Neuropsychology for clinical practice: etiology, assessment, and treatment of common neurological disorders. American Psychological Association, Washington DC
Rao S M 1986 Neuropsychology of multiple sclerosis: a critical review. Journal of Clinical and Experimental Neuropsychology 8:503–542
Rimel R W, Giordani B, Barth J T et al 1982 Moderate head injury: completing the clinical spectrum of brain trauma. Neurosurgery 11:344–351
Rocca W A, Amaducci L A, Schoenberg B S 1986 Epidemiology of clinically diagnosed Alzheimer's disease. Annals of Neurology 19:415–424
Rothwell P M, Coull A J, Giles M F et al 2004 Change in stroke incidence, mortality, case-fatality, severity, and risk factors in Oxfordshire, UK from 1981 to 2004 (Oxford vascular study). The Lancet 363:1925–1933
Saint-Cyr J A, Taylor A E 1992 The mobilization of procedural learning: the 'key signature' of the basal ganglia. In: Squire L R, Butters N (eds) Neuropsychology of memory, 2nd edn. Guilford Press, New York
Sano M, Stern Y, Williams J et al 1989 Coexisting dementia and depression in Parkinson's disease. Archives of Neurology 46:1284–1286
Schiffer R B, Kurlan R, Rubin A et al 1988 Parkinson's disease and depression: Evidence for an atypical affective disorder. American Journal of Psychiatry 145:1020–1022
Schneider L S, Olin J T, Pawluczyk S 1993 A double-blind cross over pilot study of l-deprenyl (selegeline) combined with cholinesterase inhibitor in Alzheimer's disease. American Journal of Psychiatry 150:321–323
Selby M J 2000 Overview of neurology. In: Groth-Marnet G (ed) Neuropsychological assessment in clinical practice: a guide to test interpretation and integration. John Wiley, New York
Shalat S L, Seltzer B, Pidock C et al 1987 Risk factors for Alzheimer's disease: a case-control study. Neurology 37:1630–1633
Skilbeck C 2003 The neuropsychology of vascular disorders. In: Halligan P W, Kischka U, Marshall J C (eds) Handbook of clinical neuropsychology. Oxford University Press, Oxford
Smart T 2001 Human body. Dorling Kindersley, London, p 334
Soukup V M, Adams R L 1996 Parkinson's disease. In: Adams R L, Parsons O A, Culbertson J L et al (eds) Neuropsychology for clinical practice: eitiology, assessment, and treatment of common neurological disorders. American Psychological Association, Washington DC
Sprengelmeyer R, Young A W, Calder A J et al 1996 Loss of disgust perception of faces and emotions in Huntington's disease. Brain 119:1647–1665
Stacy J, Jancovik J 1992 Differential diagnosis of Parkinon's disease and the Parkinon's plus syndromes. Neurologic Clinics 10:341–359

Starkstein S E, Brandt J, Folstein S et al 1988 Neuropsychological and neuroradiological correlates in Huntington's disease. Journal of Neurology, Neurosurgery and Psychiatry 51:1259–1263

Starkstein S E, Preziosi T J, Bolduc P L et al 1990 Depression in Parkinson's disease. Journal of Nervous and Mental Disease 178:27–31

Starkstein S E, Mayberg H S, Leiguarda R et al 1992 A prospective longitudinal study of depression, cognitive decline, and physical impairments in patients with Parkinson's disease. Journal of Neurology, Neurosurgery and Psychiatry 55:377–382

Stevenson J M, King J H 1987 Neuropsychiatric aspects of epilepsy and epileptic seizures. In: Hales R E, Yudofsky S C (eds) Textbook of neuropsychiatry. American Psychiatric Press, Washington

Strange P G 1992 Brain biochemistry and brain disorders. Oxford University Press, Oxford

Tang M, Jacobs D, Stern Y et al 1996 Effect of oestrogen during menopause on risk and age at onset of Alzheimer's disease. The Lancet 348:429–432

Teasdale G, Jennet B 1974 Assessment of coma and impairment of consciousness: a practical scale. The Lancet 2:81–84

Tennant A 1995 The epidemiology of head injury. In: Chamberlain M A, Neuman V, Tennant A (eds) Traumatic brain injury rehabilitation: service, treatments and outcomes. Chapman and Hall, London

Terry R D, Katzman R 1983 Senile dementia of the Alzheimer type. Annals of Neurology 14:497–506

Thompson P, Shorvon S 1997 The epilepsies. In: Greenwood R, Barnes M, McMillan T et al (eds) Neurological rehabilitation. Psychology Press, Hove

Trimble M R, Thompson P J 1986 Neuropsychological aspects of epilepsy. In: Grant I, Adams K M (eds) Neuropsychological assessment of neuropsychiatric disorders. Oxford University Press, Oxford

Tröster A I 1998 Assessment of movement and demyelinating disorders. In: Snyder P, Nussbaum P (eds) Clinical neuropsychology: a pocket handbook for assessment. American Psychological Association, Washington DC

Tröster A I, Paolo A M, Lyons K E et al 1995 The influence of depression on cognition in Parkinson's disease: a pattern of impairment distinguishable from Alzheimer's disease. Neurology 45:672–676

Warlow C P 1998 Epidemiology of stroke. The Lancet 352(suppl 111):14

Warlow C P, Dennis M S, Gijn J van et al 1996 Stroke: a practical guide to management. Blackwell Science, Oxford

Whitlock F A, Siskind M M 1980 Depression as a major symptom of multiple sclerosis. Journal of Neurology, Neurosurgery, and Psychiatry 43:861–865

Whittaker J N, Benveniste E N 1990 Demyelinating diseases. In: Pearlman A L, Collins R C (eds) Neurobiology of disease. Oxford University Press, New York

Will R G, Ironside J W, Zeidler M et al 1996 A new variant of Creutzfeldt-Jakob disease in the UK. The Lancet 347:921–925

Will R G, Zeidler M, Stewart G E et al 2000 Diagnosis of new variant Creutzfeldt-Jakob disease. Annals of Neurology 47:575–582

Williamson D J, Scott J G, Adams R L 1996 Traumatic brain injury. In: Adams R L, Parsons O A, Culbertson J L et al (eds) Neuropsychology for clinical practice: etiology, assessment, and treatment of common neurological disorders. American Psychological Association, Washington DC

FURTHER READING

Stringer A Y 1996 A guide to adult neuropsychological diagnosis. F A Davis, Philadelphia

Williams A C 1999 Patient care in neurology. Oxford University Press, New York

Other disorders

7

OVERVIEW

In the previous chapter we looked at the symptoms associated with the more common disorders of the central nervous system. We will turn our attention now to some of the less frequently encountered syndromes and signs that can occur in isolation or as part of a symptom complex.

Frequently, the disorders listed here form aspects of other disorders. For example, the alien hand syndrome can be observed in cases of cerebrovascular accident (CVA). Others, however, represent primary diagnoses around which other symptoms are often clustered. For example, Tourette's syndrome is often associated with attentional deficits.

This list of other disorders, however, is not meant to represent an exhaustive catalogue and only scratches the surface of what is a much greater and wider set of neuropsychological and neuropsychiatric presentations. I hope, nevertheless, to both provide the reader with a flavour of the depth, breadth and variety of the more common features of these less common disorders and present a resource wherein some of the more unusual aspects of neuropsychological symptomatology are referenced.

ALIEN HAND SYNDROME

One of the most unusual disorders to be observed in neuropsychology, the alien hand syndrome or as it is also known, the anarchic hands or diagnostic apraxia, describes a condition whereby one of the patient's hands appears to act autonomously (Biran & Chatterjee 2004). The action of the hand is involuntary and outside the patient's control. Almost always, it is the left hand that is affected, although it can be found rarely in the right hand, and sometimes the condition affects the lower limbs.

Unlike somatoparaphrenia (see below), where ownership of the affected limb is rejected, patients suffering with alien hand syndrome feel that the limb is their own, but that it will not obey them, seeming to have its own personality, and making complex, purposeful and independent movements. The level of behavioural complexity demonstrated by such patients varies from the very simple to the intricate. Perhaps, therefore, the best way to illustrate this phenomenon is to provide some examples.

There are, of course, the simple actions of the affected hand, which can include the uncomplicated grasping of nearby objects (Banks et al 1989), the unbuttoning of a shirt by the left hand after buttoning by the right (Bogen 1985), or the movement of a cup of coffee towards the patient by the right hand that is then pushed away again by the left hand (Gottlieb et al 1992). More complex actions include reversal (for example cooking with the left hand when the right hand had previously been used) and the grasping of the throat by the patient's left hand during sleep (Banks et al 1989).

Typically, alien hand syndrome is produced by a lesion to the corpus callosum or, less frequently, with involvement of the parietal and posterofrontal cortex and subcortical structures. Commonly caused by infarcts or corticobasal degeneration (Fisher 2000), alien hand syndrome has been observed in CVA, Alzheimer's disease and as a symptom in some cases of Creutzfeldt-Jackob disease (CJD) (MacGowen et al 1997).

Unfortunately, there is no cure for alien hand syndrome; however, some cases resulting from CVA resolve over time. Treatment for the disorder generally consists of attempts to occupy the affected hand with repetitive motor tasks, the utilization of relaxation techniques, or the control of the limb using spoken commands.

ANOSAGNOSIA AND ANOSODIAPHORIA

Derived from the Greek and meaning loss of knowledge, anosagnosia is the denial of a deficit or the failure to recognize the severity of a deficit. It was first described by the French neurologist Babinski in 1914 and, initially, was thought to involve a lack of awareness with regard to hemiplegia. However, it has also been described in relation to other disorders including aphasia, amnesia, apraxia, hemianopia, and cortical blindness, where it is referred to as Anton's syndrome.

Anosagnosia appears to be more common with damage to the right cerebral hemisphere (Cutting 1978) and, particularly, the right parietal lobe. However, the condition has also been described in association with a number of other cortical and subcortical structures, including the frontal lobe, temporal lobe, occipital lobe, thalamus and basal ganglia.

Anosodiaphoria is similar to anosagnosia but reflects an indifference to or lack of concern rather than frank denial with regard to a deficit or impairment. Again, this disorder was described by Babinski (1914), tends more commonly to affect the right cerebral hemisphere (Stone et al 1993), and is typically associated with excessive jocularity or unwarranted optimism.

In the past, these disorders of awareness were often viewed as a form of psychological denial or avoidance, or a stoical attempt to minimize the impact of illness, rather than representing a function of damage to the brain. Indeed, at first glance, it can still be very difficult to distinguish between an organic or functional process. However, emotionally or psychologically mediated mechanisms tend to be accessible to psychotherapeutic interventions. Anosagnosia and anosodiaphoria, on the other hand, are not.

In addition, the presence of such disorders of awareness are, of course, a barrier to rehabilitation and pose a very real problem for the members of the care team attempting to involve the patient in treatment. For, if the patient is unaware or indifferent to their particular deficit, then it is extremely difficult to engage that individual in a course of therapy that may, ultimately, have an impact.

CONFABULATION

Derived from the Latin 'confabulatus' meaning to talk together, confabulation is the unintentional filling of gaps in memory through the fabrication of information. Responses from patients that are confabulating can appear detailed, fluent, and, importantly, plausible. However, the responses of these patients can also seem bizarre and frequently do not have an obvious relationship to the topic of conversation.

As previously stated, however, confabulation is unintentional. It is, therefore, not the same as lying. Though there may be embellishment or distortion of actual events, distortion of the temporal sequence of events, or the simple invention of information, the patient does not deliberately manufacture this information but rather fills in the blanks left by a memory disorder.

Confabulation, therefore, is often associated with the type of memory disturbance frequently observed in chronic alcohol abuse, traumatic brain injury and dementia (Demery et al 2001). It is particularly associated with damage to the frontal lobes and not to be mistaken for the deliberate guessing regarding past events that some patients with memory disturbances engage in as a compensation strategy.

DELUSIONAL MISIDENTIFICATION

Capgra's syndrome or the delusion of doubles is the delusional belief that impostors have replaced individuals close to the sufferer. Usually, patients believe that an impostor has taken over the body of someone familiar to them or that they have been replaced by an exact double. Typically, the substituted individual has some sort of sinister intent and this can lead to aggression on the part of the sufferer (Thompson & Swann 1993).

The disorder has been associated with right cerebral hemisphere injuries and frontal lesions and it has been suggested that Capgra's syndrome is related to the cognitive mechanism linking emotional recognition and facial recognition (Ellis & Young 1990).

Frégoli's syndrome, on the other hand, involves the belief that persons not familiar to the patient have been invaded by a person familiar to them in order to achieve some malevolent goal. Again, this disorder has been associated with neurological abnormalities involving the right frontal and temporal regions and has been observed after traumatic brain injury (Feinberg et al 1999) as well as being associated with schizophrenia.

Reduplicative paramnesia involves the claim by the patient that they are in two or more places at one time or that the current environment is in a different location to where it is in objective reality. Usually, the location of the environment has some past or contemporary personal significance to the sufferer and the belief is persistent, despite evidence to the contrary. Again, it is seen more frequently in right cerebral hemisphere injuries and there is often involvement of the frontal and/or temporal lobes (Kapur et al 1988).

DEPRESSIVE PSEUDODEMENTIA

Also known as the depression syndrome of dementia or simply pseudodementia, depressive pseudodementia (DP) is a form of major depression that mimics the cognitive changes associated with organic dementia but is, in fact, a manifestation of a psychological disturbance. It has been suggested that as many as 10 to 20% of patients are misdiagnosed as suffering with either an organic dementia rather than depression or depression masquerading as an organic dementia (DesRosier 1992).

Unsurprisingly, in the elderly, depression is relatively common. Typically, the sources of these emotional disturbances relate to restrictions of functionality with encroaching age, the presence of an increasing number of medical conditions, and the death of loved ones and other contemporaries that serve to highlight the proximity of mortality.

In the elderly, then, major depression may be a common cause of dementia-like symptoms (Reding et al 1985). It has been suggested that the disorder occurs more frequently in women with a past psychiatric history of depression and that it is associated with a catastrophic reaction to the losses incurred in later life in those with predisposing personality characteristics (Hepple 2004).

Importantly, this form of cognitive impairment, therefore, comes under the heading of reversible dementia – a condition that, with appropriate treatment, will remit without producing the characteristic progression associated with the organic dementias. It should also, however, be remembered that DP can be extremely difficult to differentiate from an organic dementia in the early stages, and that the presence of depression alone does not exclude the patient from suffering another disorder.

To illustrate, many patients with a pre-existing dementia may also become depressed, aggravating their cognitive deficits and making the process of diagnosis much more complicated. Depression may also be the first sign of a dementing process. It is also true to say that the presence of DP does not eliminate the possibility that patients may also present with a co-existing cerebral disorder that might render some components of their impairments reversible while leaving others fixed.

Notwithstanding these observations, however, it is recognized that patients with DP tend to differ from those with organic dementias in a number of important ways. Patients with DP tend to demonstrate an abrupt onset of difficulties and the course of the illness is usually more rapid and uneven. Typically, patients are more aware of their deficits and more frequently complain of memory disorder. Often there is a pre-existing psychiatric history. Frequently, there is a question of cooperation with neuropsychological testing associated with apathy. There tend to be no neurological symptoms associated with the condition, such as dysphasia or dyspraxia, and computed tomography (CT), magnetic resonance imaging (MRI) and electroencephalography (EEG) results tend to be normal for the patient's age.

In contrast, patients with organic dementias tend to demonstrate a more insidious onset for their difficulties, with a slower and more progressive decline observed. Often there is no previous psychiatric history and limited awareness of deficit, with few complaints of memory difficulty. Typically, the patient's cooperation with neuropsychological testing is good, while other neurological symptoms can be found with increased frequency. CT, MRI, and EEG investigations often demonstrate abnormalities.

Nevertheless, differential diagnosis of the disorder remains extremely difficult and can still lead to misdiagnosis if the underlying, organic process is an atypical one, such as with CJD (Azorin et al 1993). Indeed, pharmacological and psychotherapeutic treatment for the depressive component of the condition and the ongoing monitoring of the cognitive component of DP remain the only reliable means to confirm its presence.

EPISODIC DYSCONTROL SYNDROME

Also known as intermittent explosive disorder, episodic dyscontrol syndrome (EDS) is characterized by sudden, unpredictable outbursts of explosive and sometimes violent anger and aggressive behaviour. Generally, the episode is out of proportion to the events that trigger it and irreversible once initiated. EDS differs from anger and/or temper outbursts in that it is inappropriate in degree to the inciting trigger and typically cannot be managed in the more usual manner.

It has been proposed that EDS has a neurological component. It may represent an entity similar to seizure activity and has been associated with minimal brain dysfunction (Drake et al 1992). In terms of aetiology, EDS has been linked to infections (Dolan & Kamil 1992), head trauma (Woody 1988), and epilepsy (Woermann et al 2000).

Often the condition can be misdiagnosed as a psychological disturbance. Yet, because EDS is primarily a neurological problem, psychotherapeutic intervention is of little value. Medication, however, can be helpful in the control of the condition. For example, the anticonvulsant carbamazepine has been found to be a useful treatment (Lewin & Sumners 1992).

FOREIGN ACCENT SYNDROME

This very rare condition is characterized by patients beginning to speak with an accent foreign to their natural speech. For example, a useful illustration of this disorder is the often related World War II case of the Norwegian woman who, in 1941, suffered a brain injury after being struck by shrapnel. Thereafter, she experienced language difficulties and began to speak with what was perceived to be, by those hearing her, a German accent. As a result, it was assumed that she was sympathetic to the Germans and she was ostracized by members of her local community.

Although rare, foreign accent syndrome (FAS) is generally not associated with other speech disorders such as aphasia or dysarthria. As such, FAS appears only to affect accent and does not appear to produce other problems with utterances, such as problems with syntax. It has been observed in cases of head trauma, CVA (Blumstein et al 1987) and even MS (Bakker et al 2004), suggesting a neurological basis for the disorder.

However, while a subcortical basis for the disorder has been suggested (Carbary et al 2000), causing the character of verbal expression to be changed, it seems likely that the misinterpretation of accent is in the mind of the listener. Thus, irregular speech characteristics in the prosodic speech patterns of the speaker are identified as a foreign accent by the listener.

METAMORPHOSIA AND THE ALICE IN WONDERLAND SYNDROME

Metamorphosia is a term encompassing visual, auditory or somatosensory domains and concerns: stimuli that either appear distorted (dysmorphosia), larger (macropsia) or smaller (micropsia) than they are; auditory stimuli that seem louder or softer than are; or objects or body parts that feel apparently deformed or lighter/heavier than they actually are.

Sometimes observed as an hallucinatory state associated with schizophrenia and hallucinogenic intoxication, metamorphosia, along with impairments to the sense of the passage of time (Cau 1999), forms part of the symptom complex known as Alice in Wonderland syndrome (so called because of its similarity to the distortions experienced by Alice in Lewis Carroll's novel).

This syndrome has been associated with epilepsy (Zwijnenburg et al 2002), Epstein-Barr virus infection (Cinbis & Aysun 1992), chickenpox infection (Soriani et al 1998), migraine headache (Evans & Rolak 2004) and it has even been suggested that the ingredients of a cough syrup have been responsible for its manifestation (Takaoka & Takata 1999). In terms of neurological injury, metamorphosia is thought to occur more frequently with damage to the right cerebral hemisphere and insults that involve the occipital and parietal lobes.

Interestingly, micropsia and macropsia have also been recently cited as a possible cause for the common illusion that the full moon appears larger when near the horizon than it does when higher up in the sky.

PHANTOM AND SUPERNUMERARY LIMBS

Phantom limb describes the phenomenon whereby the sufferer continues to feel the existence of an amputated body part. As such, the phenomenon can include numerous body parts such as hands, arms, legs, feet, breasts, etc. and the affected body part need not necessarily have been amputated. For example, cases of the phantom limb phenomenon have also been reported in patients experiencing congenital abnormalities and, thus, an absence of a limb (Saadah & Melzack 1994) or with damage to the spinal cord.

In many cases, sufferers also experience pain in the phantom limb as well as sensations of movement and coordination with the rest of the body. Over time, many sufferers experience 'telescoping' where the phantom limb gradually feels as if it is absorbed back into what remains of the limb and, in some cases, the phantom limb may disappear altogether.

Although, there is, as yet, no firm agreement on the causation of phantom limb sensations, it has been proposed that one of the more likely mechanisms underlying the phenomenon is a disturbance of the body's schema (a cognitive model that represents our knowledge about the arrangement of body parts and their spatial relationship to objects in the environment). Thus, a re-organization of the sensory cortex, taking place after the amputation of a particular body part, causes neurons that were previously responsive to the now missing body part to become stimulated by the remaining inputs.

Treatments for the pain arising in many cases of phantom limb are, on the whole, of only limited use and range from the use of anticonvulsant and antidepressant medication to surgical intervention; from biofeedback and acupuncture to electroconvulsive therapy (Rasmussen & Rummans 2000).

In contrast to the phantom limb phenomenon is the supernumerary limb phenomenon. In these rarer cases, patients report experiencing an additional limb such as an extra arm or an extra leg. Often such reports are associated with damage to the parietal lobe and anosagnosia may be an accompanying symptom. However, supernumerary limbs have also been known to occur briefly as a result of simple partial seizures (Riddoch 1941).

NON-EPILEPTIC ATTACK DISORDER

Also known as pseudoepilepsy, psuedoseizures and psychogenic seizures, non-epileptic attack disorder (NEAD) describes paroxysmal episodes that outwardly appear to be epilepsy. However, these episodes are not associated with the electrographic features observed in epilepsy and no other physical cause for their manifestation can be found, for example hypocalcaemia.

NEAD, therefore, is considered not to be neurological in origin but evidence of a psychological disturbance. A prompt identification of the disorder can, therefore, help to improve patient outcome through the early recognition of underlying psychological factors in presentation and a reduction in the likelihood of polypharmacy and anticonvulsant toxicity (Francis & Baker 1999).

Nevertheless, NEAD can be extremely difficult to differentiate from epilepsy for a number of reasons. First, there can be a great degree of overlap between the phenomena observed in both NEAD and epilepsy. Secondly, there are occasions when EEG recordings fail to demonstrate abnormalities in cases of epilepsy. For example, in cases of simple partial seizures, simple EEG can often be normal. Similarly, if the epileptic focus is within deep structures of the brain or the frontal cortex, EEG recordings can fail to provide evidence of electrical abnormality. Thirdly, some sufferers of epilepsy can also demonstrate NEAD. Differentiation between NEAD and epilepsy, then, is undertaken very cautiously and it may be a combination of factors that help to determine diagnosis.

Being vigilant of the above observations, then, the diagnosis of NEAD follows the exclusion of multiple causative factors. That is to say, the NEAD diagnosis results from a failure to isolate evidence for epileptic seizures through intensive investigation and, as the case for epilepsy is weakened, so there is a consequent strengthening of the case for NEAD.

To illustrate, NEAD might be suspected if an atypical epilepsy presentation is forthcoming; for example, if seizures have a long period of onset, if the ictal episodes are of a long duration, or if there is reaction to external stimuli during the event. However, it should be recalled, with reference to Chapter 6, that the range of epileptic presentation can be extremely variable and unusual. Atypicality, therefore, cannot be considered solely diagnostic for NEAD.

Historical factors might also be of use in the case evaluation of NEAD. For example, NEAD appears to be more common in females than males, and there may be a history of psychiatric disorder (Bowman & Markand 1996), emotional trauma, and/or physical/sexual abuse (Reillyet al 1999). There may also be obvious evidence of secondary gain.

As previously stated, EEG recordings can provide further evidence of NEAD as the electrical discharges one might expect to see in epilepsy are absent. However, it must be clearly understood that, once again, such findings are not diagnostic as conventional EEG can be confounded by other factors. For instance, fontal lobe epilepsy can produce some quite bizarre and less stereotypical behavioural features than is associated with other ictal events. Nonetheless, the electrical discharges associated with the disturbance can be at such a depth within the frontal lobe that simple EEG will not be able to detect it.

Another means of investigating NEAD is to look for changes in serum prolactin or to examine neuron-specific enolase levels following an episode. Prolactin levels rise with hippocampal stimulation (Trimble 1978) serving, therefore, as an indicator of ictal activity. Neuron-specific enolase, meanwhile, acts as an indicator of neuronal injury (DeGiorgio et al 1996) and can, therefore, be elevated after certain epileptic seizures. Thus, prolactin and neuron-specific enolase levels can help to strengthen the suspicion of NEAD. However, it should be remembered that these changes are, again, not necessarily good single markers for NEAD. To illustrate, increased prolactin levels are not specific to epilepsy and can be found in cases of hypotensive syncope, while conversely, prolactin levels may remain normal after status epilepticus.

Neuroimaging may also be of limited use in differentiating NEAD from epilepsy by way of visualizing neurological damage that could be the source of electrophysiological abnormalities. However, even the most sophisticated imaging techniques may lack the resolution to detect very small lesions and there are many epilepsy sufferers who have apparently normal scans.

Finally, repeated EEG, telemetric EEG and video telemetry can also prove useful in the isolation of NEAD. Such monitoring provides a great deal of useful data that single instance recording and observation cannot reproduce.

Overall, then, given the nature of the disorder and the numerous difficulties it presents diagnostically, NEAD remains a complex and delicate condition to isolate. It is, essentially, a diagnosis which, by its very nature and the ever expanding limits of our knowledge, must remain tentative. It should be based on the accumulation of evidence from a variety of sources that contradicts the diagnosis of epilepsy and never be assumed on the basis of limited observations and investigations.

POST-CONCUSSIONAL SYNDROME

Post-concussional syndrome (PCS) is a gradually self-resolving condition, not uncommon in cases of mild to moderate head injury. However, PCS does not appear to be associated with any specific biophysical markers. It has, therefore, been the source of much dispute and while there does appear to be some organic basis for the condition (Robertson 1988) there is still a great deal of argument as to the relative contribution of psychogenic and physiogenic factors (Jacobson 1995) in its development.

It manifests itself through a number of neuropsychological sequelae, including: increased frequency of headache, dizziness, diplopia, blurred vision, attentional deficit, short-term memory disturbance, reduced speed of cognition, fatigue, sleep disturbance, increased irritability, depression, anxiety, loss of confidence and emotional lability.

In general, these symptoms are transient and gradually remit, and sufferers regain a level of functioning consistent with their premorbid status. However, the presence of such symptomatology in the period before its resolution can often prove distressing for sufferers and their families, and can serve to interfere with normal occupational, academic and social pursuits.

Generally, in those individuals continuing to exhibit persistent PCS symptomatology following an injury of this nature, gradual resolution of cognitive and psychosocial deficit is usually expected to continue for up to 12 months post-trauma. It should be noted, however, that there are cases where PCS symptoms persist for longer periods and progress is often complicated by a number of contributing pre-, peri- and post-traumatic aetiological variables, such as: age, general health, psychological constitution, pre-existing psychosocial difficulty, severity of injury and so on.

REVERSIBLE DEMENTIA

Also referred to as secondary dementia, reversible dementia (RD) is not the result of a primary loss of cortical or subcortical function. Rather, as its name implies, it is a secondary process accompanying other conditions, which may be reversible with treatment (Rabins 1983). The two most common causes of RD are depression (see above under depressive pseudodepression) and reactions to medication. However, the list of other potential causes is still extensive, emphasizing the importance of a detailed history in each case of suspected dementia (Hoffman et al 1998).

Some of the causes of RD include:

- *Physical*: neoplasm, trauma normal pressure hydrocephalus; metabolic conditions such as hyponatraemia, hypernatraemia hypopituitarism, hypoglycaemia, hyperadrenalism, thyroid disease, hepatic failure, renal failure; and nutritional disorders such vitamin deficiency (B_{12}, B_1)
- *Medication*: anaesthesia, anticholinergics, anticonvulsants, antihypertensives, anxiolytics, antiarrhythmias, and anticonvulsants, etc.
- *Chemical*: alcohol or other intoxicant abuse, heavy metals poisoning, exposure to industrial agents such as organic solvents or insecticides

- *Infection*: meningitis, neurosyphilis, cryptococcus, cerebral abscess
- *Psychiatric*: chronic schizophrenia, depression (see above under depressive pseudodementia), hypomania, repeated electroconvulsive therapy
- *Environmental*: sensory deprivation.

SOMATOPARAPHRENIA

Somatoparaphrenia, a variant form of anosagnosia (Pimental & Kingsbury 1989), involves the persistent denial of ownership of a body part, usually a limb. It is usually associated with neglect, involving a visual-spatial-perceptual dysfunction manifesting as neglect of one side of the body or of extra-personal space, and, again, tends to be related to right hemisphere damage (Paulig et al 2000).

Patients with somatoparaphrenia often report that a particular limb does not belong to them but to another person, that the limb is no longer there or even that the limb has undergone some sort of transformation. The patient's attitude to the affected limb is usually hostile and can manifest itself as misoplegia, a hatred of the limb.

SYRINGOMYELIA

In order to demonstrate that not all pathology stems from illness or trauma within the brain, syringomyelia (SM) is a disorder in which a cyst forms within the spinal cord. This cyst, called a syrinx, expands over time and affects the spinal cord, producing pain, weakness, and stiffness in the back, shoulders, arms or legs. There may also be headaches, loss of ability to sense extremes of temperature, sweating, a disturbance of sexual function, and disruption of bladder and bowel control.

MRI will often demonstrate the presence of the syrinx in the spinal cord while other historical features will help to determine the type of SM. For example, hydrocephalus associated with a congenital abnormality of the brain known as the Arnold Chiari malformation (Geroldi et al 1999) or arachnoiditis (Kakar et al 1997), an inflammation of the spinal cord, may produce communicating SM. In other cases, however, non-communicating SM results from trauma, meningitis, haemorrhage or tumour. SM resulting from these aetiologies will reflect the expansion of the syrinx at the site of the spinal cord damage.

In Brown-Séquard syndrome, named after the 19th Century French physiologist, SM results from damage to one-half of the spinal cord. It is characterized by ipsilateral weakness, a loss of position sense, segmental anaesthesia at the level of the lesion, and contralateral loss of pain and temperature sensation.

TOURETTE'S SYNDROME

Tourette's syndrome describes the presence of multiple vocal and motor tics. First described by Gilles de la Tourette in 1885, the condition is not diagnosed unless there is evidence of both motor and vocal features (sufferers of one or the other are described as suffering simply with a tic disorder).

The disorder involves simple or complex motor tics such as blinking, grimacing, shoulder shrugging, brow wrinkling, hopping and clapping, etc., or, at its most complex, echopraxia and copropraxia (the copying of movement and the use of obscene gestures). These motor tics are accompanied by a variety of simple or complex vocal tics; for example snorting, sniffing, coughing, groaning, and the utterance of specific words or sentences. Again with increasing complexity, these vocal tics can incorporate echolalia, pallilalia and, in some cases, coprolalia (the use of obscene language). The urge to produce these tics is very difficult for the sufferer to resist.

Attentional problems, hyperactivity and obsessive-compulsive behaviour are also associated with Tourette's syndrome. In addition, the condition can also produce a great deal of distress for sufferers and, understandably, further difficulties in social functioning.

Onset is usually before the age of 18 years and is commonly linked to an hereditary factor (Pauls 1992), although sporadically occurring cases do emerge. Imaging studies of the brains of sufferers suggest possible problems with the basal ganglia, while other research suggests a dysfunction of the dopaminergic system (Singer et al 1991), and certainly the behaviour associated with Tourette's syndrome can be aggravated or eased by the use of medications that increase or decrease the availability of dopamine. More recently, it has also been proposed that magnesium levels might also be a factor (Grimaldi 2002).

SUMMARY

We have looked briefly at a number of disorders including alien hand syndrome, anosagnosia, anosodiaphoria, confabulation, delusional misidentification, episodic dyscontrol syndrome, foreign accent syndrome, metamorphosia and the Alice in Wonderland syndrome, phantom limb syndrome, pseudodementia, non-epileptic attack disorder, post-concussional syndrome, somatoparaphrenia, syringomyelia, and Tourette's syndrome. This very brief foray into the more unusual neurobehavioural aspects of brain dysfunction by no means represents the full spectrum of conditions that one might come across. However, it does provide an important introduction to the need to assess each case with an eye to differential analysis and also the great variety of symptoms encountered.

REFERENCES

Azorin J M, Donnet A, Dassa D et al 1993 Creutzfeld-Jakob disease misdiagnosed as depressive pseudodementia. Comprehensive Psychiatry, 34:42–44

Babinski J 1914 Contribution a l'etude des troubles mentaux dans l'hemiplegie organique cerebrale (anosagnosia). Revue Neurologique 1:845–847

Bakker J I, Apeldoorn S, Metz L M 2004 Foreign accent syndrome in a patient with multiple sclerosis. Canadian Journal of Neurological Sciences 31:271–272

Banks G, Short P, Martinez A J et al 1989 The alien hand syndrome: clinical and post mortem findings. Archives of Neurology 46:456–459

Biran I, Chatterjee A 2004 Alien hand syndrome. Archives of Neurology 61:292–294

Blumstein S E, Alexander M P, Ryalls J H et al 1987 On the nature of the foreign accent syndrome: a case study. Brain and Language 31:215–244

Bogen J E 1985 Split-brain syndrome. In: Vinken P J, Bruyn G W, Klawans H L (eds) Handbook of clinical neurology, 2nd edn. Oxford University Press, New York

Bowman E S, Markand O N 1996 Psychodynamics and psychiatric diagnoses of pseudoseizure subjects. American Journal of Psychiatry 153:57–63

Carbary T J, Patterson J P, Snyder P J 2000 Foreign accent syndrome following a catastrophic second injury: MRI correlates, linguistic and voice pattern analyses. Brain and Cognition 43:78–85

Cau C 1999 The Alice in Wonderland syndrome. Minerva Medica 90:397–401

Cinbis M, Aysun S 1992 Alice in Wonderland syndrome as an initial manifestation of Epstein-Barr virus infection. British Journal of Ophthalmology 76:316

Cutting J 1978 Study of anosagnosia. Journal of Neurology, Neurosurgery and Psychiatry 41:548–555

DeGiorgio C M, Gott P S, Rabinowiscz A L et al 1996 Neuron-specific enolase, a marker of acute neuronal injury, is increased in complex partial status epilepticus. Epilepsia 37:606–609

Demery J A, Hanlon R E, Bauer R M 2001 Profound amnesia and confabulation following traumatic brain injury. Neurocase 7:295–302

DesRosier G 1992 Primary or depressive dementia: psychometric assessment. Clinical Psychology Review 12:307–343

Dolan J D, Kamil R 1992 Atypical affective disorder with episodic dyscontrol: a case of Von Economo's disease (encephalitis lethargica). Canadian Journal of Psychiatry 37:140–142

Drake M E, Heitter S A, Pakalnis A 1992 EEG and evoked potentials in episodic-dyscontrol syndrome. Neuropsychobiology 26:125–128

Ellis H D, Young A W 1990 Accounting for delusion misidentifications. British Journal of Psychiatry 157:239–248

Evans R W, Rolak L A 2004 The Alice in Wonderland syndrome. Headache 44:624–625

Feinberg T E, Eaton L A, Roane D M et al 1999 Multiple Fregoli delusions after traumatic brain injury. Cortex 35:373–387

Fisher C M 2000 Alien hand phenomena: a review with the addition of six personal cases. Canadian Journal of Neurological Sciences 27:192–203

Francis P, Baker G A 1999 Non-epileptic attack disorder (NEAD): a comprehensive review. Seizure 8:53–61

Geroldi C, Frisoni G B, Bianchetti A et al 1999 Arnold-Chiari malformation with syringomyelia in an elderly woman. Age and Aging 28:399–400

Gottlieb D, Robb K, Day B 1992 Mirror movements in the alien hand syndrome. American Journal of Physical Medicine and Rehabilitation 71:297–300

Grimaldi B L 2002 The central role of magnesium deficiency in Tourette's syndrome: causal relationships between magnesium deficiency, altered biochemical pathways and symptoms relating to Tourette's syndrome and several reported comorbid conditions. Medical Hypotheses 58:47–60

Hepple J 2004 Conversion pseudodementia in older people: a descriptive case series. International Journal of Geriatric Psychiatry 19:961–967

Hoffman M Jeck, Kappos L 1998 Reversible dementia. Schweizerische Rundschau fur Medizin Praxis 87:773–777

Jacobson R R 1995 The post-concussional syndrome: physiogenesis, psychogenesis and malingering. An integrative model. Journal of Psychosomatic Research 39:675–693

Kakar A, Madan V S, Prakash V 1997 Syringomyelia – a complication of meningitis. Case report. Spinal Cord 35:629–631

Kapur N, Turner A, King C 1988 Reduplicative paramnesia: possible anatomical and neuropsychological mechanisms. Journal of Neurology, Neurosurgery and Psychiatry 51:579–581

Lewin J, Sumners D 1992 Successful treatment of episodic dyscontrol with carbamazepine. British Journal of Psychiatry 161:261–262

MacGowen D J, Delanty N, Petito F et al 1997 Isolated myoclonic alien hand as the sole presentation of pathologically established Creutzfeldt-Jakob disease: a report of two patients. Journal of Neurology, Neurosurgery and Psychiatry 63:404–407

Paulig M, Weber M, Garbelotto S 2000 Somatoparaphrenia: a positive variant of anosagnosia for hemiplegia. Nervenarzt 71:123–129

Pauls D L 1992 The genetics of obsessive compulsive disorder and Gilles de la Tourette's syndrome. Psychiatric Clinics of North America 15:759–766

Pimental P A, Kingsbury N A 1989 Neuropsychological aspects of right brain injury. Pro-Ed, Austin, Texas

Rabins P V 1983 Reversible dementia and the misdiagnosis of dementia: a review. Hospital and Community Psychiatry 34:830–835

Rasmussen K G, Rummans T A 2000 Electroconvulsive therapy for phantom limb pain. Pain 85:297–299

Reding M, Haycox J, Blass J 1985 Depression in patients referred to a dementia clinic: a three year prospective study. Archives of Neurology 42:894–896

Reilly J, Baker G A, Rhodes J et al 1999 The association of sexual and physical abuse with somatization: characteristics of patients presenting with irritable bowel syndrome and non-epileptic attack disorder. Psychological Medicine 29:399–406

Riddoch G 1941 Phantom limbs and body shape. Brain 64:197–222

Robertson A 1988 The post-concussional syndrome then and now. Australian and New Zealand Journal of Psychiatry 22:396–402

Saadah E S, Melzack R 1994 Phantom limb experiences in congenital limb-deficient adults. Cortex 30:479–485

Singer H S, Hahn I S, Moran T H 1991 Abnormal dopamine uptake sites in postmortem striatum from patients with Tourette's syndrome. Annals of Neurology 30:558–562

Soriani S, Faggioli R, Scarpa P 1998 Alice in Wonderland syndrome and varicella. Pediatric Infectious Disease Journal, 17:935–936

Stone S P, Halligan P W, Greenwood R J 1993 The incidence of neglect phenomena and related disorders in patients with acute right or left hemisphere stroke. Age and Aging 22:46–52

Takaoka K, Takata T 1999 Alice in Wonderland syndrome and lilliputian hallucinations in a patient with a substance-related disorder. Psychopathology 32:47–49

Thompson A E, Swann M 1993 Capgra's syndrome presenting with violence following heavy drinking. British Journal of Psychiatry 162:692–694

Trimble M R 1978 Serum prolactin in epilepsy and hysteria. British Medical Journal 2:1682

Woermann F G, van Elst L T, Koepp M J et al 2000 Reduction of frontal neocortical grey matter associated with affective aggression in patients with temporal lobe epilepsy: an objective voxel by voxel analysis of automatically segmented MRI. Journal of Neurology, Neurosurgery and Psychiatry 68:162–169

Woody S 1988 Episodic dyscontrol syndrome and head injury: a case presentation. Journal of Neuroscience Nursing 20:180–184

Zwijnenburg P J, Wennink J M, Laman D M et al 2002 Alice in Wonderland syndrome: a clinical presentation of frontal lobe epilepsy. Neuropediatrics 33:53–55

FURTHER READING

Lezak M D 1995 Neuropsychological assessment, 3rd edn. Oxford University Press, Oxford

Stringer A Y 1996 A guide to adult neuropsychological diagnosis. F A Davis, Philadelphia

Neurotoxicology

8

OVERVIEW

In the preceding chapters we have concentrated on structural pathology while only briefly touching on the effects of toxic substances on the brain. In this chapter, however, we will concentrate more specifically on the neurophysiological results and neuropsychological symptoms of exposure to a number of agents, such as pesticides, metals and solvents. We will also look at the effects of exposure to the more familiar recreational intoxicants such as alcohol, cannabis and cocaine.

The catalogue of substances able to exert an influence on the central nervous system (CNS) is very long indeed and includes agents that are both poisonous at all levels and in all forms and those whose impact changes with the level and form in which they are encountered. These range from those substances we know to be extremely toxic, such as cyanide, the more exotic and less frequently encountered toxins, such as tetrodotoxin (the extremely dangerous neurotoxin present in Puffer fish), to those that may be encountered occupationally, such as organophosphates, or those encountered recreationally, such as caffeine.

Generally speaking, the adverse effects of exposure vary with the substance encountered. Thus, there is no definitive pattern of neuropsychological symptomatology. However, while there is no specific profile to the deficits observed, it is usually the case that the symptoms produced by exposure tend to be more diffuse.

In addition, one may be able to distinguish between acute and chronic exposure or make a reasonable deduction as to the route through which the toxic substance has entered the body. For example, the symptoms of acute and chronic exposure for many substances are different; while assessment of an individual who has attempted suicide through the breathing of exhaust fumes can largely dispense with entry routes such as ingestion, skin absorption or injection and go immediately to consideration of the inhalation of carbon monoxide gas.

Obviously, with all of this in mind, this single chapter cannot review all of the toxins and the variety of presentations produced by them. What follows, therefore, is a brief description of some of the more frequently encountered substances and their behavioural and cognitive effects.

METALS

Lead

Although lead poisoning in the UK is now relatively rare, cases still appear from time to time (Elliot et al 1999). As a heavy metal, lead occurs frequently within the environment. However, it serves no physiological purpose.

Individual exposure to lead can take many forms. Until recently, lead was an additive in petrol, spread to the environment through combustion and although this has now been removed, it still remains in use in Eastern Europe. Lead-based paints, although a recognized source for potential toxic exposure, are still, however, a significant problem. Often, lead poisoning is associated with older paint sources and the ingestion of paint fragments by children. Lead can also be found in some older water supply systems where pipes, valves and soldered joints can contain the metal. Finally, the industrial use of lead is also a potential exposure route as the material is still used in a great number of products including production of lead batteries (Lai et al 1997) and ceramic glazes (Kawai 1976).

Through its interference with protein synthesis, a number of neurotransmitters and the development of synaptic connections within the brain, lead is able to exert an influence on brain development, leading to long-term difficulties for children exposed to the toxin. In addition, lead is also freely able to cross the placenta in pregnancy. Gestational lead poisoning is, therefore, not only a risk for mothers but also to the developing fetus (Shannon 2003).

Lead can produce both acute and chronic effects and, although the incidence of poisoning has been greatly reduced by efforts to remove lead in commercial use and prevent its release into the environment (Juberg et al 1997), exposure can still occur, giving rise to a number of different behavioural and cognitive symptoms. These symptoms, of course, vary with the level and duration of exposure and include: anaemia, persistent headache, vomiting, abdominal pain, forgetfulness, fatigue, apathy, agitation, increased irritability, mood changes, reduced motor speed and muscle weakness. Also, as exposure levels increase, symptoms include an increase in the weakness of extensor muscles leading to wrist drop and foot drop, paralysis, hallucinations, delirium, seizures, coma and finally death.

Mercury

Made famous by the behaviour of the Mad Hatter in Lewis Carroll's book *Alice in Wonderland*, Mad Hatter's syndrome was observed amongst 19th Century workers who were exposed to mercury in the felt hat industry. Mercury occurs in three different forms: inorganic salts, organic compounds and metallic mercury, each causing different physiological effects. The inorganic mercury salts irritate the gut and can cause severe kidney damage. Organic mercury compounds are able to cross the blood–brain barrier and, thus, cause damage to the brain. Metallic mercury, meanwhile, is again able to cross the blood–brain barrier, causing significant problems. However, metallic mercury may also be converted to organic mercury by bacteria, and in this form enter the food chain, as was the case at Minimata Bay in Japan in the 1950s (Langford & Ferner 1999).

Again, toxic exposure can occur in a variety of ways. Mercury is used in the production process of a number of items, from thermometers to X-ray machines and paper to electrical equipment. Mercury has even been used as a preservative in some latex-based paints (Agocs et al 1990). In some places in the world, mercury is also used in pesticides and fungicides, with the possible result of contamination of crops and, as with the case of poisoning observed at Minimata Bay, mercury can enter the body through the ingestion of contaminated fish.

Contamination of the environment has also occurred in other areas of the world; for example, China, the Philippines, Siberia, and South America, where both historic and ongoing mining practices rely on mercury amalgamation for gold extraction, giving rise to high levels of the substance in plant and animal life in the area (Eisler 2004). Mercury has also been found to be a constituent in some cosmetic products, causing large scale exposure problems (Sin & Tsang 2003), and it has also been implicated in certain traditional and religious healing practices. Possible exposure to the mercury vapours from the amalgam used by dentists has also been cited as a possible source of contamination and, although this remains controversial, some studies do suggest that the low-level, repeated exposure of dentists and dental workers to mercury may need to be monitored (Ritchie et al 2002).

The symptoms of mercury toxicity vary with the level of exposure and the type of substance encountered. In acute cases, where death does not occur through respiratory, renal or gastrointestinal dysfunction, a number of symptoms may be encountered. For example, metal fume fever is characterized by fatigue, weakness, fever, dizziness, headache, abdominal pain, dyspnoea and dysuria. Similarly, acrodynia, characterized by a rash, generalized pain, excessive sweating and increased heart rate tends to be observed in children. Meanwhile, erethism, characterized by increased irritability, excitability, anxiety, insomnia, and social withdrawal tend to be observed in cases of chronic exposure.

With exposure to inorganic mercury, one might expect the development of a tremor, fatigue, irritability, excess salivation, motor weakness, pain, vomiting, diarrhoea, renal failure, vertigo, nystagmus, blurred vision, a reduced visual field, optic neuritis and atrophy, an impact on visuospatial abilities, progressive personality change, mood fluctuation, and insomnia.

Organic mercury, on the other hand, causes peripheral neuropathy, ataxia, tremor, paraesthesia, cortical blindness, a reduction in the visual fields, deafness, dysarthria, excessive sweating and salivation, fasiculations, and a reduced speed of cognition and poor memory. Sometimes those exposed will report a metallic taste in the mouth. Some cases will also demonstrate a brown mark or line on the teeth.

Aluminium

Being one of the most prevalent elements on earth, it is not surprising that traces of aluminium can often be found in many food stuffs and water supplies. In normal circumstances this is not a matter for concern. However, if the concentration of aluminium exceeds the body's capacity to excrete the substance, then it can accumulate in various bodily tissues causing illness and even death.

Acute cases of exposure are rare. However, in those with impaired renal function the accumulation of this metal can result in a number of symptoms. Indeed, aluminium has been implicated in patients undergoing kidney dialysis (Savory et al 1985) who can suffer with a condition known as dialysis dementia (dialysis encephalopathy).

A link between exposure to aluminium and the development of the neurodegenerative condition Alzheimer's disease has also been suggested (Gupta et al 2005). However, this link remains speculative and, although important, aluminium does not yet appear to be the sole factor in the development of a number of neurodegenerative diseases. However, despite this, it has been suggested that long-term exposure is to be avoided (Campbell 2002).

In addition, there is also the case of the effects of exposure to larger quantities of aluminium. The accidental discharge of aluminium sulphate into the water supply of Camelford in Cornwall in the UK in 1988 (Owen & Miles 1995) resulted in a number of ingestion exposures to some 20 tonnes of the substance being released at a water treatment plant. Here, neuropsychological dysfunction was discovered in those exposed (McMillan et al 1993) and was later suggested to be related to cerebral dysfunction (Altmann et al 1999).

The symptoms of aluminium toxicity typically include apraxia, myoclonus, speech disorder and difficulty in swallowing. The neuropsychological presentation can include personality change and reductions in attentional functioning, memory, and executive functioning, which, if severe, can qualify as a form of dementia.

PESTICIDES AND INSECTICIDES

Given that these chemicals are meant to be lethal to some forms of life, it is not perhaps surprising to find that they can also be responsible for toxic effects in humans. The most frequently encountered and widely used of these are the organophosphates (OPs). Originally, these substances were produced as an insecticide. However, because of their properties affecting neuromuscular transmission, they were later developed during World War II as neurotoxic weapons. Today, OPs are still extensively used as insecticides, although it should be recalled that the terrorist attack in the subways of Tokyo in 1995 relied on a substance known as sarin, which is a member of the OP group.

OPs act by inhibiting acetylcholinesterase, resulting in an increase of acetylcholine throughout the nervous system. This results in a number of physical symptoms. However, it has also been suggested that the effects of chronic, low-dose exposure are primarily neuropsychological.

Exposures to OP tend to be either occupational or environmental. Occupational exposure to OPs occurs amongst agricultural workers, industrial workers and pest control workers. Environmental exposure includes contact with residential pesticides used by residents or pest control workers or when a domicile or public area lies adjacent to an agricultural site using OPs. It should be borne in mind also that domestic or environmental exposures may also pose a greater risk in that there is also a lack of protective equipment such as breathing masks, etc. (Morrow 1998).

OP administration has even been seen as a source of poisoning in cases of homicide (De Letter et al 2002) and has been suggested as a factor in genetic damage and the development of some cancers in low-dose occupational exposure (Webster et al 2002), with other studies suggesting that even domestic exposure levels could have a genetotoxic effect (Lieberman et al 1998).

Acute exposure to OPs typically results in headache, increased salivation, increased lacrimation, excessive sweating, intestinal cramps, vomiting, ataxia, fasiculations, weakness, respiratory distress, diarrhoea, pupil constriction, paraesthesia, confusion, emotional lability, fatigue and insomnia. In more extreme cases, seizures can occur secondary to anoxia. Death from exposure tends to result from cardiac or respiratory failure.

In cases of both chronic and acute exposure, a variety of cognitive and emotional disturbances may be present. These can include reduced speed of information processing, reduced motor speed, poor coordination, circumscription of memory and anxiety.

ORGANIC SOLVENTS

Organic solvents are carbon-based compounds useful in the dissolving and dispersal of non-water soluble materials, such as fats, oils, resins, rubber and plastics. This group heading includes a multitude of different chemicals, such as acetone, benzene, toluene and styrene that can be used as organic solvents. These include hydrocarbons, glycols, amines, esters, ethers and ketones. Widely used in industry and manufacturing, these substances are to be found in many paints, varnishes, lacquers, thinning agents, adhesives, and cleaning and degreasing agents and are also used in the production of certain dyes, printing inks, textiles and plastics.

This very widespread use means that we may come into contact with organic solvents through a wide variety of household and commercial products and that, as a result, exposures may be of a mixed variety. That is to say that exposure may involve more than one substance.

Industrial exposures in those working with these substances are not difficult to account for (e.g. Linström 1981), but environmental exposures may also occur if an individual lives close to an industrial plant where these substances are used and may accidentally contaminate water supplies or the soil, be released into the air, or enter food.

Some exposures occur as a result of deliberate action on the part of the individual. Organic solvents may be inhaled or 'sniffed' when an individual recreationally inhales paints, glues, thinners, etc., to produce euphoria, excitement, sedation, delusions, and visual and auditory hallucinations (Miller & Gold 1991).

The symptoms of contact with various organic solvents can vary widely with the individual and some variation will occur with the agent involved. However, generally, contact is characterized by chronic or acute exposure, and low or high-level dose intensity.

Acute exposure usually involves complaints of nausea, headache, fatigue, dizziness, poor attention and concentration, confusion, and disorientation. In some cases there may be gait disturbance, coordination problems, respiratory difficulties and irritation of the skin. Increasing intensity of exposure is accompanied by a loss of consciousness, paralysis, seizure and finally death associated with respiratory or cardiovascular arrest.

In those cases where exposure is the result of the deliberate act of inhaling fumes from petrol, glues, paints and thinning agents, etc. for recreational purposes, symptoms can also include a feeling of intoxication, euphoria, and hallucination. In neuropsychological terms, such exposures can also result in widespread cognitive impairments and physical symptoms that can persist long after exposure or even, in some cases, prove to be irreversible.

Chronic exposure to low doses may present with a slower onset of symptoms and, in many cases, may be difficult to associate with organic solvent contact. In cases where occupational exposure is suspected, patients may demonstrate an intermittent pattern of difficulties reminiscent of their working patterns. To illustrate, they may have fewer or no symptoms when not working at the weekends. Patients may complain of headache, fatigue, insomnia, dizziness, paraesthesia, personality change, emotional lability, depression, memory dysfunction, poor attention and concentration, and reduced speed of information processing.

GASES

Carbon monoxide

Carbon monoxide (CO) is a colourless, odourless gas produced by the burning of materials containing carbon. CO is, therefore, a byproduct of combustion from numerous sources and household appliances including cigarettes, motor vehicle engines, portable heaters, gas-fired water heaters, charcoal grills, paraffin-fuelled space heaters, etc. Most often, CO exposure occurs as a result of faulty or obstructed ventilation or as a consequence of suicide attempts. However, its source can also be extremely unusual as was the case when it was implicated as the source of contamination following the use of explosives at a construction site near a residential area (Auger et al 1999).

Typically, CO causes problems through its higher affinity for haemoglobin than oxygen. Thus, where oxygen should bind to the haemoglobin in our blood, CO competes to form carboxyhaemoglobin more efficiently. This results in relative anaemia, having a profound impact on those tissues requiring a great deal of oxygen, with the resultant depression of cardiac functioning and hypotension causing further difficulties.

The early diagnosis and treatment of CO exposure can be quite difficult as the associated symptoms can often mimic other vague complaints such as a flu-like illness (Harper & Croft-Baker 2004). However, a tell-tale sign might be that the patient's skin appears very pink because the CO binding to haemoglobin causes light to be shifted to the red end of the spectrum.

In acute cases, patients may complain of headache, drowsiness, fatigue, apathy, breathlessness, chest pain, palpitations, nausea, vomiting, diarrhoea, weakness, confusion and syncope. There may even be visual disturbances, memory problems, seizures, and coma. Chronic cases of CO exposure, on the other hand, may also present with these symptoms but also demonstrate gradually evolving neuropsychiatric problems and frank impairments of cognitive functioning. In either case, exposure, particularly if prolonged or of higher intensity, can lead to irreversible brain damage resulting in persistent neuropsychological difficulties.

Phosgene

Phosgene, also known as carbonic dichloride, carbon oxychloride, and carbonyl dichloride, can exist as both a highly toxic gas or in a liquid state. First discovered by Sir Humphrey Davy in the 19th century by passing carbon monoxide and chloride through charcoal, phosgene was developed during World War I with chlorine gas as a battlefield weapon.

Today, although it may still be considered to be a possible threat in terms of chemical warfare (Karalliedde et al 2000), phosgene has more industrial uses. Occupational exposure, therefore, is the more likely source (e.g. Wyatt & Allister 1995).

It is used in the production of a number of items including polycarbonate resins, polyurethane, aniline dyes, some pesticides, and certain pharmaceuticals. It is also used in the production of glass as a bleaching agent for sand and in the uranium enrichment process. Phosgene can also be produced by the heating or burning of a number of household products containing chlorinated organic compounds, such as carbon tetrachloride, chloroform and methylene chloride. These include solvents, paint removers, and dry cleaning fluids.

Classified as a pulmonary irritant, the symptoms of phosgene exposure include headache, weakness, breathlessness on exertion, light-headedness, cough, chest pain, irritation of the eyes and increased lacrimation, irritation of the nasal passages, irritation of the throat, and anxiety. Where the skin or the clothes are wet there may also be burning of the skin as the phosgene breaks down to form hydrochloric acid.

Phosgene can be toxic at relatively low concentrations and even short exposure to relatively low concentrations of the gas can be lethal. Death from exposure is typically related to pulmonary problems and secondary hypoxia, although it can also occur secondary to laryngospasm with greater exposures.

RECREATIONAL DRUGS

Thus far we have briefly examined some of the effects of exposure to a number of metals, pesticides, organic solvents, and gases, some of which are encountered occupationally and some of which can be encountered environmentally. However, there are also groups of substances that individuals voluntarily expose themselves to or abuse. Some of these substances represent justifiable uses, for example as medications; some of these are classified as recreational and vary in the legality of their use; for example caffeine is used by many people while heroin is not.

In this section, then, we will look more closely at some of these substances. We will not, however, widen our study to include the toxic effects of medication, such as the benzodiazepines or phenothiazines, as these are comprehensively dealt with in other freely available publications, such as the British National Formulary (Dinesh 2005). This is not to say that such exposures are not considered to be an important factor in neuropsychological assessment, only that other texts are able to provide more detailed information.

Alcohol

One of the most widely abused substances, alcohol can produce significant neuropsychological effects in both acute exposure cases and with more chronic use. Similarly, different patterns of neuropsychological performance are associated with different kinds of alcohol use. Alcohol, like many other substances, has a depressive effect on the CNS. Its ingestion not only affects CNS function directly but also, through secondary biological mechanisms, produces a series of metabolic events that, in turn, can have an effect on functioning.

Many of us have experienced the intoxicating effects of alcohol when taking the substance recreationally in social circumstances. These, of course, vary with the level and form in which the alcohol is taken. They can include a reduction in motor speed, poorer coordination, a reduction in memory functioning, a drop-off in verbal skills, reduced speed of cognition, a reduction in mental flexibility and a mild tendency to perseverate. The result of such consumption is generally reversible and the after-effects of such exposure is limited.

However, with more frequent consumption of a higher dose level, combined with other risk factors, comes an increased risk of dependency and more dramatic neurological and neuropsychological impairment. Chronic alcoholism is associated with a profile of cognitive performance suggesting persistent difficulties with learning, memory, executive functioning, visuospatial ability and motor functioning.

Wernike-Korsakoff's disease or syndrome may be observed in those cases where malnutrition and/or liver disease associated with a long history of chronic alcohol abuse causes a vitamin B_1 (thiamine) deficiency (Allen & Landis 1998). Symptoms include ataxia, ocularmotor problems and confusion. If treatment of this problem is undertaken, then the great majority of sufferers will survive. However, most of them will demonstrate difficulties characterized by significant problems with memory, planning abilities and organizational skills. Interestingly, such is the density of the memory problem that early on, many sufferers begin to confabulate in order to fill the obvious gaps in their knowledge. In general, such individuals lack insight into their condition and many become apathetic, resulting, in many cases, in a lack of further interest in alcohol.

The question of a distinct form of widespread cognitive impairment known as persistent alcoholic dementia remains debatable (Allen & Landis 1998).

However, when it has been described it is typically associated with a long history of alcohol abuse and is characterized by an extensive cognitive, emotional and personality functioning decline. In such cases a widespread cerebral atrophy is observed; however, in addition to memory problems, patients with this diagnosis also demonstrate significant difficulties with skills associated with the frontal lobes.

Caffeine and nicotine

Both caffeine and nicotine produce a stimulatory effect on the human body. Caffeine is the most widely used psychostimulant in the world (Evans & Griffiths 1999) and acts by increasing dopamine levels in the frontal areas of the brain. Nicotine, on the other hand, whilst also having an effect on dopamine, stimulates the endocrine system.

Caffeine is, of course, available from many dietary sources. Drinks such as coffee and tea contain this stimulant but it is also available in many soft drinks such as cola beverages. It is even to be found in chocolate. In normal use, the stimulant properties of caffeine promote cognitive arousal and reduce fatigue levels. It can increase alertness and the ability to concentrate, and in lower doses is rarely a problem. At higher doses, however, caffeine can produce a number of less pleasant symptoms such as anxiety, excitability, tachycardia, cardiac arrhythmia, duiresis, gastrointestinal disturbance, psychomotor agitation and insomnia. Finally, cessation of caffeine use after prolonged, heavy usage can result in headache, fatigue, drowsiness, anxiety and depression.

Nicotine, meanwhile, promotes the release of hormones acting at various sites within the brain This results in an increase in alertness and arousal, greater efficiency in terms of cognitive processing, a reduction in fatigue and a sedative action reducing anxiety and inducing mild euphoria.

Nicotine also has an effect on the availability of dopamine and serotonin and exerts an influence on the stress hormones, indirectly stimulating the release of opioids in the system. Thus, nicotine also directly and indirectly acts upon the brain's reward mechanisms promoting further use of the substance. Increasing doses results in acute nicotine poisoning with symptoms including nausea, vomiting, increased salivation, sweating, abdominal pain and diarrhoea.

Cannabis

Cannabis, although apparently coming to the fore during the 1960s, has in fact been used for many years and early historical accounts of its use abound. Today it is still one of the most widely used recreational drugs but has also become a treatment for certain conditions such as glaucoma and is being studied in relation to multiple sclerosis. Containing tetrahydrocannabinols (THCs), cannabis can be inhaled or ingested, although inhalation when the drug is smoked represents the swiftest means of introducing the substance into the body.

Again the symptoms of use can be divided into acute or chronic categories. The acute effects of the drug can produce euphoria and feelings of well-being, relaxation, grandiosity, drowsiness, changes in the perception of the passage of time, perceptual alterations, poorer coordination, and impairment of attentional skills, problem solving and judgement. It can also increase appetite, a condition termed colloquially as the 'munchies'.

Cannabis, despite the popular belief that it only induces a euphoric or relaxed state, can also produce more negative changes such as depression, suicidal ideation, anxiety, panic, paranoia, depersonalization and even psychosis (Semple et al 2005). At higher dose levels there may be also memory impairment, disorientation, and changes in perception giving rise to illusions and hallucinations.

Chronic use may also produce diminished social, occupational and academic drive resulting in an amotivational syndrome (Kumar & Clark 2005). However, while the effects of cannabis can be observed to linger for some hours or days after its use, there appears to be little evidence of long-term residual cognitive deficit (Iversen 2005).

Ecstasy

Methylenedioxymethamphetamine (MDMA) or as we more commonly know it, ecstasy, is derived from amphetamine. It has become increasingly popular in the last two decades, chiefly because of the belief that it is a 'safe' drug inducing feelings of euphoria, disinhibition and empathy. However, the substance was first created in the early part of the 20th century and experimented with by the USA military during the 1950s. Later still, during the 1970s, the drug was experimented with again as having possible psychotherapeutic uses. It was, however, during the 1980s and 1990s that MDMA use became widespread as profitability amongst the young became a factor.

MDMA acts by altering neurotransmitter levels and, in particular, it selectively affects the release of serotonin (Mathias et al 2000). In animal studies, MDMA has been observed to cause damage to serotonin-producing sites in the brain (Schmued 2003). Nevertheless, there are, as yet, no human equivalent studies. However, it is possible that, as the drug is metabolized by the liver, and certain members of the population do not possess the liver enzyme responsible for metabolizing MDMA, some of the deaths associated with exposure might be related to this. In addition, while MDMA is relatively easily synthesized, it is often poorly produced and mixed with other substances such as heroin, leading to additional problems.

Often the symptoms of negative MDMA reactions or overdose can be difficult to clarify. This is because the social setting for drug use is typically in an environment that means that other drugs such as alcohol, cannabis, cocaine and heroin are also available. However, symptoms can generally include hyperthermia, increased heart rate, palpitations, increased blood pressure, chest pain, nausea, vomiting, urinary retention, headache, blurred vision, ataxia, insomnia, anxiety, agitation, paranoia and seizures. As a result of increased blood pressure there is also a risk of stroke. In the longer term there may also be complications through residual mood changes, attentional and memory problems and even liver damage, although this is still under study.

It is also interesting to note that the psycho-emotional effects of MDMA, which one might think would produce an increased libido, conversely appear to impair sexual drive and functioning. Indeed, recent research suggests that the state produced by MDMA may be akin to the postorgasmic state and that the drug impairs sexual responses through the possible alteration of the substance prolactin (Passie et al 2005).

Cocaine

Like caffeine and nicotine, cocaine is a stimulant. However, not only is it more potent than either of these, it is also both highly addictive and associated with a number of neurological disorders. Derived from the coca leaf, cocaine was used by some native populations to reduce the effects of fatigue. Today it can be smoked or inhaled/snorted nasally. It can also be taken by injection subcutaneously or intramuscularly, as was the case with the Arthur Conan Doyle character, Sherlock Holmes. This form of administration is, however, only rarely used as it slows absorption of the drug.

Whatever the route into the body, cocaine acts by stimulating the CNS through the modification of neurotransmitter uptake and metabolism, affecting dopamine, serotonin, noradrenaline (norepinephrine) and acetylcholine levels. Cocaine also has a local anaesthetic effect caused by a direct effect on tissues blocking nerve impulses.

The symptoms of cocaine exposure can be divided into acute and long term. The acute effects of the drug include euphoria, a sense of well-being and restlessness (Anderson 1994). There is also a reduction in fatigue, increased heart rate, increased blood pressure, increased alertness and arousal. In early use it can also act as an aphrodisiac. However, in the longer term, cocaine use is often associated with insomnia, depression, suicidal ideation, aggression, paranoia and hallucinations, and the drug can actually reduce libido and even produce impotence.

Seizures can also occur with cocaine use (Enevoldson 2004) and may not be limited to long-term users as it is associated also with those who have not tried the drug before. The great majority of these seizures are single, generalized events and are not linked to permanent neurological impairments. However, in some cases, particularly in chronic users, there may be cerebral atrophy and electroencephalogram (EEG) abnormalities suggesting that the seizures may be the result of the structural changes of long-term exposure. Cocaine is also associated with acutely increased blood pressure. This, in combination with other over-stimulation of the CNS, may also lead to an increased risk for haemorrhagic stroke (Enevoldson 2004).

Toxic exposure or overdose in cocaine use is characterized by hyperthermia, seizure and coma. Death usually ensues as a result of cardiac or respiratory failure or from hyperthermia.

Cocaine may also play a role in certain movement disorders and can also have a secondary influence on cardiac and vascular systems resulting in the development of disorders such as thrombosis and myocardial infarction. Pregnant mothers using cocaine also have a higher rate of spontaneous abortions and premature births, and the babies of cocaine users may develop cerebral infarcts, seizures and microcephaly (an abnormally small head).

SUMMARY

In this chapter we have concentrated more specifically on the effects of a number of toxic agents including some metals, pesticides, gases and solvents. We have also taken a closer look at the effects of some recreational substances including alcohol, caffeine, nicotine, cannabis, ecstasy and cocaine. Such detailed observation demonstrates that not only are there structural, traumatic and progressive pathological conditions to be considered in an individual's neuropsychological status but also a host of occupational, environmental and recreational substances that are also able to exert their own influence over functioning.

REFERENCES

Agocs M M, Etzel R A, Parrish R G et al 1990 Mercury exposure from interior latex paint. New England Journal of Medicine 323:1096–1101

Allen D N, Landis R K 1998 Neuropsychological correlates of substance use disorders. In: Snyder P, Nussbaum P (eds) Clinical neuropsychology: a pocket handbook for assessment. American Psychological Association, Washington DC

Altmann P, Cunningham J, Dhanesha U et al 1999 Disturbance of cerebral function in people exposed to drinking water contaminated with aluminium sulphate: retrospective study of the Camelford water incident. British Medical Journal 319:807–811

Anderson R M 1994 Practitioner's guide to clinical neuropsychology. Plenum Press, New York

Auger P L, Levesque B, Martel R et al 1999 An unusual case of carbon monoxide poisoning. Environmental Health Perspectives 107:603–605

Campbell A 2002 The potential role of aluminium in Alzheimer's disease. Nephrology Dialysis Transplantation 17(suppl 2):17–20

De Letter E A, Cordonnier J A, Piette M H 2002 An unusual case of homicide by use of repeated administration of organophosphate insecticides. Journal of Clinical Forensic Medicine 9:15–21

Dinesh M (ed) 2005 British national formulary, vol 49. Pharmaceutical Press, Oxon

Eisler R 2004 Mercury hazards from gold mining to humans, plants, and animals. Reviews of Environmental Contamination and Toxicology 181:139–198

Elliot P, Arnold R, Barltrop D et al 1999 Clinical lead poisoning in England: an analysis of routine sources of data. Occupational and Environmental Medicine 56:820–824

Enevoldson T P 2004 Recreational drugs and their neurological consequences. Journal of Neurology, Neurosurgery and Psychiatry 75:9–15

Evans S M, Griffiths R R 1999 Caffeine withdrawal: a parametric analysis of caffeine dosing conditions. Journal of Pharmacology and Experimental Therapeutics 289:285–294

Gupta VB, Anitha S, Hegde M et al 2005 Aluminium in Alzheimer's disease: are we still at a crossroad? Cellular Molecular Life Sciences 62:143–158

Harper A, Croft-Baker J 2004 Age and Aging 33:105–109

Iversen L 2005 Long-term effects of exposure to cannabis. Current Opinion in Pharmacology 5:69–72

Juberg D R, Kleiman C F, Kwon S C 1997 Position paper of the American Council on Science and Health: lead and human health. Ecotoxicology and Environmental Safety 38:162–180

Karalliedde L, Wheeler H, Maclehose R et al 2000 Possible immediate and long-term health effects following exposure to chemical warfare agents. Public Health 114:238–248

Kawai M 1976 Urinary non-precipitable lead in lead workers. British Journal of Industrial Medicine 33:187–192

Kumar P, Clark M 2005 Clinical medicine 6th edn. Elsevier Saunders, Edinburgh

Lai J S, Wu T N, Liou S H et al 1997 A study of the relationship between ambient lead and blood lead among lead battery workers. International Archives of Occupational and Environmental Health 69:295–300

Langford N, Ferner R 1999 Toxicity of mercury. Journal of Human Hypertension 13:651–656

Leiberman A D, Craven M R, Lewis H A et al 1998 Genotoxicity from domestic use of organophosphate pesticides. Journal of Occupational and Environmental Medicine 40:954–957

Linström K 1981 Behavioral changes after long-term exposure to organic solvents and their mixtures: determining factors and research results. Scandinavian Journal of Work and Environmental Health 7(suppl 4):48–53

McMillan T M, Freemont A J, Herxheimer A et al 1993 Camelford water poisoning accident: serial neuropsychological assessments and further observations on bone aluminium. Human and Experimental Toxicology 12:37–42

Mathias E L, Mathias R S, Gamma A et al 2000 Psychological and physiological effects of MDMA ('ecstacy') after pre-treatment with the 5-HT2 antagonist ketanserin in healthy humans. Neuropsychopharmacology 23:396–404

Miller NS, Gold MS 1991 Organic solvent and aerosol abuse. American Family Physician 44:183–189

Morrow L A 1998 Neurotoxicology. In: Snyder P, Nussbaum P (eds) Clinical neuropsychology: a pocket handbook for assessment. American Psychological Association, Washington DC

Owen P J, Miles D P 1995 A review of hospital discharge rates in a population around Camelford in North Cornwall up to the fifth anniversary of an episode of aluminium sulphate absorption. Journal of Public Health Medicine 17:200–204

Passie T, Hartmann U, Schneider U et al 2005 Ecstasy (MDMA) mimics the post-orgasmic state: impairment of sexual drive and function during acute MDMA-effects may be due to increased prolactin secretion. Medical Hypotheses 64:899–903

Ritchie K A, Gilmour W H, Macdonald E B et al 2002 Health and neuropsychological functioning of dentists exposed to mercury. Occupational and Environmental Medicine 59:287–293

Savory J, Bertholf R L, Wills M R 1985 Aluminium toxicity in chronic renal insufficiency. Clinics in Endocrinology and Metabolism 14:681–702

Schmued L C 2003 Demonstration and localization of degeneration in the rat forebrain following a single exposure to MDMA. Brain Research 974:127–133

Semple D M, McIntosh A M, Lawrie S M 2005 Cannabis as a risk factor for psychosis: systematic review. Journal of Psychopharmacology 19:187–194

Shannon M 2003 Severe lead poisoning in pregnancy. Ambulatory Pediatrics 3:37–39

Sin K W, Tsang H F 2003 Large-scale mercury exposure due to a cream cosmetic: community-wide case series. Hong Kong Medical Journal 9:329–334

Webster L R, McKenzie G H, Moriarty H T 2002 Organophosphate-based pesticides and genetic damage implicated in bladder cancer. Cancer Genetics and Cytogenetics 133:112–117

Wyatt J P, Allister C A 1995 Occupational phosgene poisoning: a case report and review. Journal of Accident and Emergency Medicine 12:212–213

FURTHER READING

Albers J W, Berent S 2005 Neurobehavioural toxicology: neuropsychological and neurological perspectives. Psychology Press, New York

Hartman D E 1988 Neuropsychological toxicology: identification and assessment of human neurotoxic syndromes. Pergamon Press, New York

Recovery

9

OVERVIEW

Thus far, we have looked at how the central nervous system (CNS) is organized, its structure and function, and some of the pathological mechanisms underlying damage. In this chapter, our aim is to consider the neurophysiological and neuropsychological features of recovery and to examine some of the individual factors that influence this process.

Perhaps, the most frequently repeated question to be heard in neuropsychological treatment is: 'How long will it take for me to get better?' Sadly, the often repeated response to this question is another question: 'How long is a piece of string?' Such a response, far from being an attempt to intellectually divert patients from a more global assessment of recovery, actually underscores the limitations that many of us working with brain injury have for long-term prediction of outcome.

In short, in each case there are numerous variables to consider and the simple answer to the question of when and how much recovery will take place is that we do not know. Each individual will present with a different profile of components that will each play a role in overall recovery. These components include the type of injury, site of injury, medical history, age, sex, handedness, premorbid psychological constitution, the presence of comorbidity, emotional response, access to rehabilitative treatment, financial situation, and so on; the list is almost endless.

Thus, each case must be carefully assessed with regard to the relative influence of each of these biopsychosocial factors and general judgement of the issues of both short-term and long-term outcome discussed in terms of generalities rather than specifics. This allows recovery to take place at its own pace and within its own limits, rather than placing what are often arbitrary restrictions on a complex and, as yet, still poorly understood process.

So, in answer to the question of how long a piece of string is, we could reply, twice the distance from the middle to end! An answer which, although correct, simplifies the puzzle, embraces generality, and allows the individual piece of string to be the final arbiter of its own length.

MECHANISMS OF DAMAGE

The biological mechanisms underlying recovery are, as we have already observed, poorly understood. In the acute stages of injury to the CNS, the causative factors contributing to depressed function are most likely to include the form of insult, for example the type of mechanical trauma involved in a head injury, and the various physiological responses to it, for example oedema. Some of these factors will exert a more short-term influence, for instance metabolic depression, while some will have a more lasting effect, such as structural damage to the tissues.

The more temporary changes accompanying brain injury, in most cases, will begin to recede after a relatively short period of time. Such a process, then, would appear to restore functioning in areas previously demonstrating signs of impairment. To illustrate, a patient might demonstrate a relatively swift improvement in expressive speech skills shortly after a stroke, reflecting the diminution of cerebral oedema and return of normal metabolic activity.

Longer-term recovery, however, in the region of months or even years, cannot be understood in terms of these processes. What then are the mechanisms by which longer-term recovery takes place? In order to gain a better perspective with regard to these longer-term mechanisms of recovery, it is first necessary to develop a fuller contextual understanding of some of the degenerative events that follow injury to the brain.

Notwithstanding the various aetiological factors involved, then, damage to the brain instigates a variety of secondary physiological processes. These occur both at the site of damage and at sites more remote from the location of the insult.

At the site of damage, in addition to the structural harm done to tissues or the frank loss of tissue, necrosis occurs. Within some 24 hours, this localized death of cells is followed by the process of phagocytosis, in which astrocytes begin the removal of debris and dead cell tissue. After roughly a week, new capillaries begin to form at the site of damage.

This process of debris removal can take some time to complete and may proceed for a number of months. Finally, however, through the process of glosis, only glial cells remain, while astrocytes form a scar which, it should be noted, may itself impede the functional regeneration of remaining cells.

Meanwhile, at locations more distant from the site of direct damage, cellular degeneration can also occur, causing additional problems. The nature of this degeneration depends largely on the portion of the nerve cell damaged.

As explained in Chapter 2, neurons consist of a cell body and structural extensions known as axons and dendrites. Anterograde degeneration, also known as Wallerian degeneration after Waller, the first person to note its occurrence in the 19th century, involves the breakdown of an axon after it has been cut from the cell body. In this case the cell body remains intact but the axon dies. Retrograde degeneration, on the other hand, involves the breakdown of the cell body, dendrites and what remains of the axon after the axon is cut. In this case, the entire neuron dies.

In addition, cells that innervate or are innervated by a degenerating nerve cell can also be involved. This is termed either anterograde or retrograde transneuronal degeneration. Thus, with anterograde transneuronal degeneration, the adequate stimulation of nerve cells receiving inputs from a damaged neuron fails to be maintained and the receiving cell dies. Retrograde transneuronal degeneration, conversely, occurs when nerve cells that previously supplied stimulation to damaged neurons begin to degenerate.

The process of transneuronal degeneration may also be accompanied by calcification, where deposits of calcium accumulate. However, while the exact mechanism involved in this process is, as yet, poorly understood, these calcium deposits may be visualized on scan images of the brain, denoting certain types of CNS damage.

In addition to these cellular changes, brain damage may also be accompanied by a number of other physiological responses that will also have their effect on brain function. Oedema occurs in the brain just as it does when other portions of the body are traumatized. However, the brain is confined within the skull. Thus, the swelling of brain tissues can lead to increased intracranial pressure and consequent depression of function.

Alterations in blood flow, metabolic activity, glucose uptake and neurotransmitter levels may also cause disruption. This cascade of changes may even be accompanied by autoneurotoxicity, where the oxygen deprivation caused by certain types of damage triggers the release of an excitatory neurotransmitter (Kolb & Whishaw 1996), which, in turn, over-stimulates the cells causing a build-up of toxic waste products resulting in cell death.

Given the nature and extent of these cellular and physiological responses, then, it will be understood that the neuropsychological prognosis, in the short term, in any given case, is somewhat rudimentary. In the intermediate term, as these processes settle or are completed, prognosis is strengthened and the prediction of functional outcomes improved.

However, the prediction of outcome, the degree of recovery, and the length of time it might take to recover are, at this stage, still very much matters of conjecture. For although population statistics and the probabilities generated therein might afford us some degree of confidence in making more general observations, individual variability will tend to render more specific judgements much more difficult. Recovery, during this phase, then, is still presented in terms of likelihoods rather than certainties.

THEORIES OF RECOVERY OF FUNCTION

To fully appreciate the numerous factors that effect recovery beyond those of the acute and intermediate stages, therefore, we must consider the various biological explanations provided. Several means have been proposed as mediating recovery in the longer term. These can be divided into three broad categories: cellular, structural and process mechanisms.

Physiological mechanisms include a number of suggested processes. However, while it can be observed in the peripheral nervous system (PNS), it will be noted that the regeneration of CNS neurons to re-establish their previous connections does not occur. Nevertheless, other cellular mechanisms may play a limited replacement role for this process.

Collateral sprouting consists of the growth of the axons of neighbouring neurons to replace lost axons, while re-routeing occurs where a neuron that has lost its target puts forth new axons to seek out new targets. It is also interesting to note that nerve growth factor (NGF), a protein produced by glial cells, has been suggested as playing a role in these mechanisms by promoting growth in damaged neurons.

Denervation super-sensitivity, meanwhile, refers to the proliferation of receptors in tissues previously innervated by damaged neurons, making them hypersensitive to remaining stimulation. The silent synapse theory, however, suggests that pre-existing but previously silent or behaviourally obscure connections may exist that become overtly active when some other part of the system is damaged.

With regard to the structural mechanisms underlying recovery, it has been suggested, although it is no longer a popular theory, that underused areas of the brain substitute for the functions of damaged areas. Similarly, vicaration suggests a substitution of the functions of damaged areas but that these functions are performed by adjacent areas of the brain. The theory of redundancy, on the other hand, suggests that the brain is possessed of back-up systems that allow neural communication to continue when other systems break down. Finally, sparing is a process whereby certain behaviours survive damage.

Process theories, however, maintain that recovery may be represented by reorganization and the development of changes in the behavioural strategies used to compensate for damage. These theories suggest either that the plasticity of the brain is such that it is able to perform limited functional reorganization, or that our brains are able to compensate for damage by performing tasks previously undertaken by a damaged area through the substitution of alternate behaviour. For example, the use of a notebook can, to one degree or another, compensate for impairment in memory.

INDIVIDUAL FACTORS IN RECOVERY

Quite apart from these more generalizable cellular, physiological and process mechanisms, there are also a number of individual variables that will affect the rate and degree of recovery. These factors can be broadly grouped into two areas: biophysical and psychological.

The biophysical aspects influencing recovery include a number of factors, some of them more easily quantifiable than others. Age at the time of injury is, perhaps, the most simple to evaluate, the general rule being that the younger the patient the quicker and more robust the recovery. Age is also a factor in the development of certain kinds of pathology. For example, younger individuals tend to suffer with head injuries, whereas a great many older patients present with stroke. In addition, older patients may exhibit signs of cognitive decline associated with the aging process that younger patients do not.

Sex is also a component that must be factored into any judgement regarding recovery. Some theories suggest a difference between the anatomical and functional structure of male and female brains that assign an advantage to females in cases of brain injury. To illustrate, it has been proposed that females are, generally, less lateralized for function than males. Damage to functions associated with a particular location within the brain might, therefore, be compensated for by remaining functional components at other locations.

It has also been observed that females tend to possess a greater number of fibres in the corpus callosum, the structure connecting the two hemispheres of the brain. Thus, according to some, females may be able to transfer information from one cerebral hemisphere to another more effectively than males. Still other research suggests that female hormones confer some degree of neuroprotection in cases of traumatic brain injury (Wagner et al 2005).

Sex, like age, also influences the development of certain conditions. For example, the sex ratio in stroke indicates that more males than females develop strokes. Similarly, males are more likely to experience traumatic brain injuries than females.

Similar to the argument that females are less lateralized for function, it has also been proposed that left-handedness is also associated with a profile of codominance in functional lateralization (Vesagas et al 1993). It has been argued, therefore, that certain cases of left-handedness are linked to a less strong lateralization of function to the left or right cerebral hemispheres. Thus, recovery may take place as a result of the action of compensatory mechanisms in an undamaged region partially responsible for function.

Neuropsychological and psychological factors in the recovery process tend to focus on premorbid cognitive ability, personality functioning and behaviour. For instance, the level of premorbid intellectual functioning is also an important factor in recovery. Generally speaking, those who possessed a higher IQ before injury will demonstrate a better outcome. This is most likely because a higher level of premorbid function resources means that a particular individual may have a greater fund of cognitive resources to bring to bear in the recovery process. It is also true to say that an individual operating at a higher than average level before an injury will tend to operate better after impairment than someone with only an average level of performance.

To illustrate, a higher than average performance of, say, 120 IQ points prior to an injury might be reduced by 20 points after injury. This would place the patient in the average range. However, an individual with a premorbid IQ score of 95 points, sustaining a similar injury and the same 20 point loss, would fall into the below average range.

Conversely, however, a higher level of premorbid functioning, while it might afford some degree of resilience in terms of brain injury, might also offer further difficulties in terms of emotional functioning and adjustment. Which is to say that, while brain injury is a potentially devastating event for all, the patient with a higher level of premorbid functioning, while they may be able to perform more efficiently postmorbidly than many of their peers, may be more aware of their impairments and exhibit more emotional difficulties such as depression.

Personality is also a significant factor to consider in recovery; however, even in the unimpaired, personality remains one of the most difficult areas to assess. Nevertheless, generally speaking, those with a more cheerful, optimistic, positive, extrovert and resilient personality will tend to demonstrate better outcomes than others.

It is also true to say that premorbid emotional tendencies will also tend to be exaggerated by injury, leading individuals with a preinjury propensity for more negative emotional reactions to demonstrate an increased frequency of these postinjury. In addition, inappropriate emotional reactions may also hamper engagement in the rehabilitation process, exacerbating problems, delaying progress and, therefore, negatively impacting on outcomes.

Finally, poor outcomes may also be evident in cases where a pattern of premorbid chronic alcohol or other intoxicant use exists. Such agents may also themselves contribute to injury. For example, excessive alcohol intake may play a role in a fall that causes a depressed skull fracture.

Given the array of elements involved in the recovery process, then, it is little wonder that it is so difficult to provide definite answers to individuals attempting to gain some perspective with regard to their particular injury or illness. Many different professionals, because of their orientation and place within the system of care, will give different estimates of the degree of recovery and the time it might take to achieve. Physicians may look at the problem in terms of physical recovery; for example the time it will take to heal a fractured bone. A neuropsychologist may look at the problem in terms of the more subtle changes noted in cognition; for example the statistical probability that memory will improve in a given time.

In both of these cases, statistical likelihood garnered from population observations will provide a guide. A physician might say that the bulk of physical recovery is observed in the first 6 months postinjury. A neuropsychologist might respond that their neuropsychometric evaluations would indicate that improvement might be expected over a period of 2 years. However, while both of these observations are correct, neither is wholly true.

In the end, while the greater part of gross recovery is exhibited in the first 6 months and may continue at a slower but still noticeable rate for a further 18 months, patients continue to report more subtle improvements in their symptoms for years after an event. The process of recovery, then, while it can be quantified in terms of the magnitude and temporal relationships for large populations, varies considerably for each individual. Any judgement of prognosis, therefore, needs to be carefully evaluated with regard to all of the above factors.

TREATMENT

Having looked at the various mechanisms involved in damage and natural recovery, we will now turn briefly to the current approaches to treatment. These fall into three categories: rehabilitation strategies, pharmacological therapies and surgical interventions.

Rehabilitation seeks to achieve an optimal level of functioning in terms of the patient's residual impairments, be these psychological, physical or environmental. Such an endeavour is most effective when a multidisciplinary team approach to treatment is taken. Such a team usually comprises a physician, neuropsychologist, speech and language therapist, occupational therapist, physiotherapist, and nursing staff (Fig. 9.1).

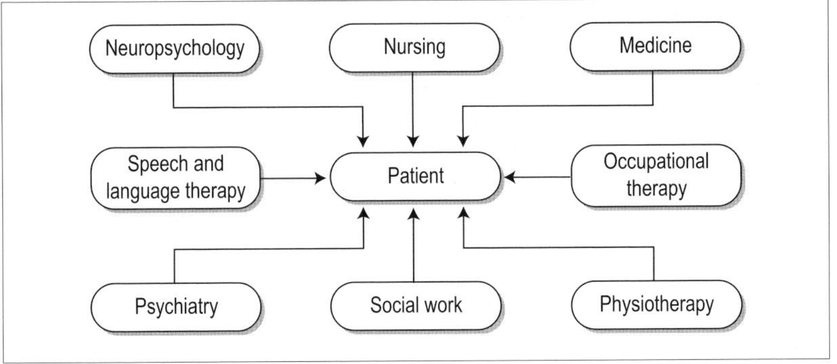

Fig. 9.1 Rehabilitation team members.

Broadly, rehabilitation interventions may be divided into those that address the patient's needs whilst still an inpatient and then those that build upon these foundations and address the patient's needs as an outpatient. Such inputs usually involve goals such as the re-establishment of self-care activities, basic motor and sensory interventions and the development of cognitive skills. Outpatient inputs include the adaptation of newly acquired inpatient compensatory skills to the wider environment, the development of new skills and strategies to meet the greater demands of the environment, assistance with reintegration, and a focus on vocational, educational or recreational endeavours.

With regard to the neuropsychological components of such rehabilitative treatments, this usually begins with a detailed assessment in order to highlight specific areas of intervention. This is followed by cognitive skills retraining in those areas demonstrating deficit and the development of strategies to aid the implementation of this new learning. Neuropsychological input should also aim to provide a forum for emotional reactions to the illness or trauma, provide a mechanism through which further team input is obtained, if needed, and attempt to deal with the concerns and questions of families and carers.

Naturally, each cognitive treatment plan is tailored to the individual needs of each patient. However, some general rules are important to remember when it comes to the rehabilitation of cognitive skills.

Stimulation in the early stages following brain injury is very important. Who among us has not heard the saying 'if you don't use it you'll lose it' and this tends to be true in terms of treatment as well. Therefore, involvement in treatment in the early stages is important for, while the brain will recover spontaneously, early therapeutic intervention can improve outcomes.

The forced use of impaired systems can also be helpful in the restoration of function. Similarly, practice in the use of an impaired system can be helpful, especially if this is surplus to requirements of what is normally required. Such repetitive training, therefore, makes use of over-learning to ensure that new skills become habitual rather than atypical adaptations.

In addition, the tasks that are to be over-learned, for example a method of memorizing complex number strings, should have some relevance to the individual's circumstances or be useful in the performance of daily activities. To illustrate, if a task or strategy does not possess features that are useful to the patient, the likelihood is that it will not be utilized. Therefore, while it may not be relevant to recall seven random numbers it may be of use to have learned a system to recall the digits in telephone numbers.

It is also important that the rehabilitative tasks provided should be broken down into simple components. This ensures that patients with compromised cognitive systems are not overloaded and that the successful completion of a given task, a potent motivator, is more likely.

Motivational factors should also be considered as contributing to overall achievement. Small improvements in functioning gained at the expense of long working periods can be frustrating. Whereas stable and consistent improvements observed over repeated shorter periods of working time reduce fatigue and frustration and encourage engagement.

Finally, it should be kept in mind that cognitive skills retraining should be continued even when an area of stability in functioning is reached. Often, levels of input reflect the levels of recovery observed. However, perseverance, even if this only results in seemingly small improvements, can help to reduce the impact of deficit over time.

Pharmacological intervention in brain injury still continues to produce mixed results, although experimental results with animals suggest that recovery rates can be increased if both pharmacological treatments and rehabilitation are combined. Nevertheless, there are some drugs licensed in the UK to treat the cognitive decline associated with Alzheimer's disease. However, these, it should be remembered, do not arrest or reverse cognitive decline, rather they delay or reduce impairment through the manipulation of neurotransmitter systems thought to be associated with cognitive deficit.

Likewise, the surgical interventions in brain damage are still, by and large, experimental. Some of these, such as the procedures involved in the control of the symptoms of Parkinson's disease, do not effect a cure but help to control manifestations of the disorder. Others, such as the transplantation of new tissues into the brains of patients suffering with certain disorders show more promise, but suffer both from difficulties with the surgical techniques required and objections to the use of, for example, fetal tissues.

FUTURE POSSIBILITIES FOR TREATMENT

What potential treatments for brain damage are on the horizon? Although it was believed that once the brain has formed and matured there is no possibility that new cells can be formed, this turns out not to be the case. There is a type of cell that populates certain areas of the brain known as subependymal cells or stem cells.

These cells have the ability to renew themselves and become new neurons, even in adults. In the future it may be possible, therefore, to take these cells from someone suffering brain damage, genetically modify them to produce neurotransmitter substances that have been lost through damage, culture and grow them outside the body and then re-introduce them into the donor without the concern of rejection.

Another possibility is nanotechnology and the development of implantable silicon-based neurons to take over the functions of damaged brain areas (Fromherz 2003), while a recent development has demonstrated the growth outside the body of neuronal tissue on carbon nanotubes (Lovat et al 2005) with applications of this technology possibly being implants to enhance neural signal transfer in cases of spinal damage.

SUMMARY

In this chapter we have examined both the physical and psychological features of the recovery process and considered some of the individual factors influencing this process. This has taken in the short-term cellular mechanisms associated with damage from phagocytosis, glosis, and the formation of scar tissue by astrocytes; the types of neuron degeneration that can occur at regions further from the site of damage; and the other physiological responses associated with injury, including oedema, changes in blood flow and changes in metabolic activity.

In addition, we have also concentrated on some of the cellular, structural and process mechanisms that might play a role in the long-term recovery of function, as well as looking at the question of the influence of individual variables, including age, sex, handedness, premorbid intellectual functioning, personality and emotion.

Finally, we have looked at some of the current treatment options with regard to brain injury, considered the basic principles of cognitive skills retraining, and examined possible future directions that intervention might take, including the use of stem cells and the development of nanotechnology.

REFERENCES

Fromherz P 2003 Neuroelectronic interfacing: semiconductor chips with ion channels, nerve cells, and brain. In: Waser R (ed) Neuroelectronics and information technology, 2nd edn. Wiley, New York

Kolb B, Whishaw IQ 1996 Fundamentals of human neuropsychology, 4th edn. W H Freeman, New York

Lovat V, Pantarotto D, Lagostena L et al 2005 Carbon nanotube substrates boost neuronal electrical signalling. Nano Letters 5:1104–1110

Vesagas T S, Lee T K, Bartham G et al 1993 Recovery from aphasia and conversion of handedness: a case report. Annals of the Academy of Medicine Singapore 22:526–528

Wagner A K, Fabio A, Puccio A M et al 2005 Gender associations with cerebrospinal fluid glutamate and lactate/pyruvate levels after severe traumatic brain injury. Critical Care Medicine 33:407–413

FURTHER READING

Herdegen T, Delgardo-Garcia J 2004 Brain damage and repair: from molecular research to clinical therapy. Kluwer Academic, Boston

Stein D G, Brailowsky S, Will B 1995 Brain repair. Oxford University Press, New York

Neuropsychological assessments

10

OVERVIEW

If the curtains are closed and you hear hoof beats outside the window, how do you know if they come from horses or zebras? The answer? Statistical likelihood. In neuropsychology, such thinking excludes the common before embracing the rare, a problem that can easily overtake the inexperienced in assessment.

To illustrate, a patient presenting with what, on the surface, appears to be a memory disorder may, in fact, be demonstrating signs of an attentional deficit which, although it impacts on memory functioning, is not a mnestic disorder per se. Thus, by carefully assessing all aspects of the system of memory and those other cognitive skills that underpin it, we are able to differentiate between attentional factors and memory factors.

In short, we are able to begin the process of excluding the zebras and accepting the horses, tentatively constructing a profile that is based on the evaluation of the simple before moving on to assessment of the complex. This is not to say that zebras do not occur. They can and sometimes do confound the assessment process. However, such instances are rare and can generally be avoided if there is careful attention to detail.

In this chapter, then, we will explore some of the more common assessment techniques, providing an overview of the more frequently encountered measures used by neuropsychologists. Such a process, it is hoped, will also help to give life to some of the observations made in previous chapters with regard to brain function, and help the reader to understand the dynamic nature of cognitive, emotional and behavioural function as it applies to the discipline of neuropsychology.

Background to assessment

What, then, is the nature of neuropsychological assessment, how does it differ from other forms of neurological investigation, and what instruments exist to help us to measure these seemingly intangible aspects of neuropsychological functioning?

Broadly speaking, neuropsychological evaluations, unlike many neurological procedures, are not invasive and do not require a physical examination of the patient. In general the neuropsychometric measures employed are called 'paper and pen' tests, seeking to understand the neurobehavioural aspects of the patient through the careful and standardized examination of their responses to verbally, visually, or somatosensorily presented stimuli.

Neuropsychologists use a great many such validated and objective tests to measure brain function. While neurological examination involves evaluation of the structural, physiological and metabolic functioning of the brain, the neuropsychological assessment remains the only reliable means to evaluate neurobehavioural function. Neuropsychological tests, then, provide a quantitative measure of functioning that can be compared with normative values, and also a qualitative appraisal of the various components of behaviour that form a part of these quantitative observations.

Such evaluations are performed for a number of reasons: to confirm or clarify a diagnosis, to define impairments and assess their impact on the individual, to provide a profile of strengths and weaknesses as a guide to rehabilitation, to monitor changes in functioning over time, to monitor the efficacy of treatment, to clarify which, if any, compensatory strategies might help to ameliorate a specific problem, or to perform research into a specific area.

On the whole, these different aims in terms of the evaluation process will, by dint of their different goals, be reflected in the testing procedures used and the choice of neuropsychological tests used. In general, neuropsychologists fall into two groups: those who administer test batteries and those who administer batteries of tests. In general, the former group applies large, fixed measurement tools to patients; while the latter group applies more flexible, single measures that are more tailored to individual patient complaints. Each method has its advantages and disadvantages, and neither is better or worse than the other.

Notwithstanding these observations, however, the essential factors of neuropsychological evaluation to keep in mind here are that: the study of brain and behaviour relationships takes place under controlled conditions; the assessment involves the administration of a comprehensive battery of standardized psychometric tests; and the evaluation will generally help to characterize the extent of how an injury, if present, specifically affects the cognitive, emotional and behavioural functioning of the patient. This is something that standard physical examinations and neuroimaging studies cannot provide.

What follows, then, is an introduction to some of the standardized batteries of tests utilized by neuropsychologists and an explanation of their use. It does not, however, represent an exhaustive list of assessment instruments as such an undertaking would fill a book in its own right. The following, therefore, is a sample of some of the more common assessment procedures that might be encountered. A fuller account of a great many more of the tests and assessments used can be found in the further reading list at the end of this chapter.

TESTS DESIGNED TO SAMPLE A RANGE OF COGNITIVE FUNCTIONS

Test instruments can be broadly divided into those that sample a wide range of cognitive functions and those that look more specifically at a single function. We will look first at some of the batteries of tests used to assess groups of functions.

Luria-Nebraska Neuropsychological Battery (LNNB)

Based around the observation that cognition consists of a dynamic process based on an array of elementary components, the Luria-Nebraska Neuropsychological Battery (LNNB) (Golden et al 1985) has its origins in the observations of the Russian neuropsychologist Alexander Luria. It offers a set of comprehensive tests designed to measure a wide range of neuropsychological functions. As such, therefore, the LNNB falls into the category of large, standardized test batteries.

Utilizing an individually calculated, critical cut-off score based on age and level of education, the LNNB was designed for use with individuals 15 years or older. It provides both an overall measure of cerebral dysfunction as well as lateralization and localization points for the assessment of deficit. In order to determine the nature and extent of both general and specific deficits, the various subtests within the battery assess a number of abilities represented on clinical scales. These include motor functions, rhythm and tactile performance, visual skills, expressive and receptive speech skills, reading and writing, arithmetic skills, memory functions and intellectual processes.

The battery itself can be administered within some 1.5 to 2.5 hours either as a whole or be spread over a number of less intensive sessions. It has the advantage of providing a great deal of useful data and has been described as a portable test; that is, it is easily administered outside the neuropsychologist's office in different environments, for example at the patients beside. However, the test is quite large and makes use of a number of test item stimuli initially making the battery quite difficult to master. The user must also to be conversant with both a great many different testing procedures as well as having an understanding of Luria's systems approach to cognitive functioning.

Personal experience with the LNNB indicates that while it can be extremely useful it also suffers from two distinct problems. First, some of the considerable number of items included on the test tend to tap cognitive skills which do not form part of the outcome measures. Secondly, the use and interpretation of the LNNB is as much an art as a science. The battery, as a whole, therefore, requires a great deal of knowledge and experience on the part of the user.

Halstead-Reitan Battery (HRB)

Again falling into the category of large, standardized batteries, the Halstead-Reitan Battery (HRB) (Reitan & Wolfson 1993) provides an impairment index score derived from performance on five tests: the category test, finger oscillation test, seashore rhythm test, speech sounds perception test, and tactual performance test. In addition to these regular measures, there are further tests that may be added to assess other factors. However, these additional procedures do not form part of the impairment index score. These additional tests include the trail-making test (which we will look at in more detail later), aphasia screening test, sensory perceptual examination, and the grip strength test.

This battery can, again, provide a large number of useful observations. It is, however, time-consuming to administer, and on the whole, while it is able to differentiate between brain-damaged patients and neurologically intact individuals, it is not as successful in differentiating brain-damaged from psychiatric patients.

Moreover, the impairment index score on the original test battery does not describe the degree of dysfunction observed. It merely provides an assessment of the likelihood that a given individual has brain damage. Nevertheless, this has, to some degree, been overcome by the use of additional subtest item analysis and the use of the average impairment ratings score as well as the general neuropsychological deficit scale.

Wechsler Adult Intelligence Scale (WAIS)

Substantially revised, reformatted and adapted over the course of some years, the Wechsler Adult Intelligence Scale (WAIS) (Wechsler 1997a) provides an assessment of a broad range of abilities and is the single most used test in neuropsychological assessment. Based on the concept that intelligence is largely abstract, the psychometric approach of the WAIS assumes that intelligence, as a general label for a group of processes that can be indirectly defined from observable behaviours and responses, is nevertheless a trait demonstrating individual differences. Thus, the WAIS, in its various forms and as it is applied in the field of neuropsychology, assumes that there is a fundamental relationship between these observable behaviours and the neurological components on which they are based.

Consisting of a number of subscales, the latest version of the instrument, WAIS-III (Wechsler Adult Intelligence Scale, 3rd edn), and its predecessors, the WAIS (Wechsler Adult Intelligence Scale), WAIS-R (Wechsler Adult Intelligence Scale Revised) and WAIS-R NI (Wechsler Adult Intelligence Scale Revised Neuropsychological Instrument) broadly assesses abilities within various cognitive domains.

Updated with the addition of new subtests and reflecting societal and cultural norms, the WAIS-III can be used with individuals between the ages of 16 and 89 years. It is divided into measures of verbal and performance skills and allows for the interpretation of a patient's global performance through an appreciation of what is called the full scale IQ.

The WAIS-III also allows for observations of verbal and performance IQs as well as providing for comparisons between the verbal and performance measures and the full scale IQ. Verbal subscales include information, similarities, comprehension, arithmetic, digit span, vocabulary and letter and number sequencing. Performance subscales include picture completion, digit-symbol coding block design, matrix reasoning, picture arrangement, symbol search, and object assembly.

In addition to the full scale verbal and performance levels of interpretation, the WAIS-III also allows for the interpretation of performance on individual subscales. Furthermore, users of the assessment are also able to calculate further scores for verbal comprehension, perceptual organization, processing speed and working memory.

Overall, the WAIS-III represents a very useful and versatile instrument that allows for a wide range of assessment and interpretation over and above evaluation of general intellectual functioning. However, the test is relatively large and can be time consuming, with administration times extending to 2 hours or more on some occasions. This can, therefore, have a detrimental effect on some patients who experience fatigue when administration is prolonged.

Wechsler Abbreviated Scale of Intelligence (WASI)

To overcome the problem of prolonged administration times and the impact these can have on a patient's performance, the Wechsler Abbreviated Scale of Intelligence (WASI) (Wechsler 1999) provides a reliable but briefer measure of intellectual functioning. For use with individuals aged 6 to 89 years, the WASI provides verbal, performance and full scale IQ scores, much like the WAIS-III (see above).

However, because the WASI provides a two subtest and a four subtest format, allowing for flexibility in administration time and degree of intensity of assessment, the test takes between 15 and 30 minutes to complete. Such a reduction enables a quick measurement of general cognitive functioning.

Clearly, the WASI is not intended as a replacement for the more detailed evaluation provided by the WAIS-III. However, it does represent a means of more swiftly assessing intellectual functioning. The only drawback to such a procedure is that there is a consequent reduction in the range of observations of functioning made.

Kaplan Baycrest Neurocognitive Assessment (KBNA)

The Kaplan Baycrest neurocognitive assessment (KBNA) (Leach et al 2000) is another comprehensive test battery examining a wide range of performance in various neurocognitive domains. It yields an index score for overall performance, as well as individual scores for performance in specific domains including attention and concentration, immediate memory, delayed recall, recognition memory, spatial processing, verbal fluency, and reasoning/conceptual shifting.

Additional portions of the battery allow for the measurement of other areas such as orientation, mental control, motor programming, selective visual attention, selective auditory attention, reading skills, auditory comprehension, praxis, emotion and expression. Scores on these subtests, however, do not go towards the calculation of the total performance score or the individual neurocognitive domain scores.

For use with those aged 20 to 89 years, the battery can be completed in around 60 minutes and offers a great deal of flexibility in terms of the various subtests included. The KBNA, therefore, allows the administrator to tailor its application to the needs of the assessment.

Repeatable Battery for the Assessment of Neuropsychological Status (RBANS)

Designed as a short screening battery providing rapid assessment of a range of cognitive functions, the Repeatable Battery for the Assessment of Neuropsychological Status (RBANS) (Randolph 1998) can be used to quickly evaluate cognitive status through the measurement of attention skills, language functioning, visuospatial/constructional abilities, and both immediate and delayed memory functioning. This makes it useful as a screening instrument in cases such as dementia, head injury and stroke when more complex test batteries might be more impractical.

The RBANS can be completed in around 30 minutes and is designed for use with those aged 20 to 89 years. It provides both a global performance score as well as a score representing the various cognitive domains sampled. Importantly, the RBANS comes in two parallel forms, the A and B versions, and, therefore, allows individuals to be repeat tested over time, reducing the effect that practice might have on their test results.

Dementia Rating Scale (DRS)

Like the WAIS-III (see above) the Dementia Rating Scale (DRS) has been substantially revised. The updated form of the test is known as the DRS-2 (Mattis et al 2002) and provides a measurement of a wide range of cognitive functioning. It has been particularly useful in the detection, assessment and monitoring of degenerative disorders but can also gauge performance in other neurological disorders.

Like the MEAMS and SIB (see below) the DRS-2 evaluates function at the lower end of the spectrum, providing scores for both overall performance and individual performance in specific areas including attention, initiation/perseveration, construction, conceptualization and memory.

Overall, the DRS-2 is a short test, taking approximately 20 minutes to administer, and can be utilized with individuals aged 55 to 89 years, providing useful observations of cognitive performance.

Middlesex Elderly Assessment of Mental State (MEAMS)

The Middlesex Elderly Assessment of Mental State (MEAMS) (Golding 1989) consists of 12 subtests assessing function in the areas of orientation, memory, learning, naming, comprehension, arithmetic, visuospatial skills, perception, fluency and motor functioning. Stimuli and tasks on the test are simpler and designed to evaluate performance in cases of significant impairment and act as a screening instrument prior to further, more detailed assessment.

Given the relative simplicity of the test, it has been used mainly to detect and assess gross cognitive dysfunction in the elderly. However, this instrument is also useful in cases where significant impairment in younger individuals makes the use of other measures impractical.

Like the RBANS (see above), the MEAMS comes in two parallel forms allowing for repeated assessment and reducing practice effects. Also, the test is relatively short and can be completed in around 10 minutes.

Severe Impairment Battery (SIB)

In a departure from tests that detect and assess the presence of neuropsychological impairments, the Severe Impairment Battery (SIB) (Saxton et al 1993) assumes the presence of a degree of impairment and is designed to assess functioning at the lower end of the performance scale. The test contains, therefore, a number of very simple tasks and is intended to evaluate performance in the areas of attention, orientation, language, memory, visuospatial skills, constructional skills, praxis and social interaction.

Taking only 20 minutes to complete, the SIB can be utilized with individuals aged 51 to 91 years. It is useful in assessing the performance of patients demonstrating severe difficulties and has, therefore, been used to assess and monitor cases of severe dementia.

TESTS DESIGNED TO ASSESS SINGLE COGNITIVE FUNCTIONS

Other tests of cognitive functioning are designed to investigate a more restricted range of abilities. They are, therefore, more sensitive to specific deficits or provide more comprehensive evaluations within a single cognitive domain.

Wechsler Memory Scale (WMS)

Like the WAIS-III, the Wechsler Memory Scale – third edition (WMS-III) (Wechsler 1997b) has been substantially revised over the course of time. Like its predecessors the WMS (Wechsler Memory Scale) and the WMS-R (Wechsler Memory Scale Revised), it offers a comprehensive evaluation of memory functioning. In addition, the WMS-III has been conormed with the WAIS-III, providing a valuable means of assessing memory with intellectual functioning.

The WMS-III provides scores for various aspects of memory functioning including auditory and visual immediate memory, a combined assessment of immediate memory, auditory and visual delayed recall, auditory recognition, general memory and working memory.

Age ranges for this test are between 16 and 89 years and, again, it provides a wealth of data with regard to individual mnestic functions. However, like the WAIS-III, the instrument as a whole can be quite time consuming, taking some 75 minutes to complete. This, of course, can be quite tiring for some individuals, raising the additional possibility of fatigue effects in test performance.

Wechsler Memory Scale – third edition abbreviated (WMS-III A)

To again overcome the problem of extended administration times and the effect that these can have on performance, the Wechsler Memory Scale – third edition abbreviated (WMS-III A) (Wechsler 2003) provides a faster means of assessing memory function than the WMS-III (see above). The test is, again, sensitive to mnestic disorders and offers an evaluation of general memory functioning as well as providing scores for immediate and delayed recall. However, being an abbreviated form, it avoids prolonged testing in situations where it is not practical to administer the full test.

Results from the test can be compared with the WAIS-III (see above) and can also be used to estimate performance were the full WMS-III to be given. The age range for this test is the same as for the full WMS-III (see above) but evaluation time is only in the region of 15 to 20 minutes.

Rivermead Behavioural Memory Test (RBMT)

Now in its second edition, the Rivermead Behavioural Memory Test (RBMT II) is a test of everyday memory functioning (Wilson et al 2003). Unlike other tests of memory, the RBMT II assesses functioning as it applies to everyday situations rather than augmenting the more traditional procedure of assessing memory in a fixed, laboratory-like manner.

The test can be used to both assess and monitor change over time and subtests consist of a number of measures used to assess memory difficulties in common situations and modalities. For example, there are test items that assess ability to remember an appointment and recall a story. The RBMT II also has a wide age range of 16 to 96 years for application and can be completed in around 30 minutes.

Test of Everyday Attention (TEA)

The Test of Everyday Attention (TEA) (Robertson et al 1994) is a measure of attentional functioning. It comes in three parallel forms and like the RBMT II (see above) largely assesses functioning through everyday situations. Subtests include measures of selective attention, sustained attention, divided attention, auditory attention and visual attention.

With an age range between 18 and 80 years, this measure takes some 50 to 60 minutes to complete and can be utilized with a number of different patient populations.

Paced Auditory Serial Addition Test (PASAT)

The Paced Auditory Serial Addition Test (PASAT) (Gronwall 1977) is a measure of sustained and divided attention, speed of information processing, flexibility, and simple arithmetic ability. It is administered via audio tape or compact disk with single digits presented every 3 seconds and the patient asked to add each new digit to the one immediately before it.

Again this is a relatively brief test to administer and can be used across a wide age range. However, the task of serial addition can be quite daunting for patients and the ensuing anxiety this produces can lead to problems with performance.

Trail Making Test (TMT)

The Trail Making Test (TMT) is a component of the HRB (see above) but acts as a stand-alone measure sensitive to the effects of central nervous system (CNS) deficit. It is a standardized visual search and sequencing task assessing attention and concentration, coordination, speed of information processing, resistance to distraction, and cognitive flexibility. It is also sensitive to a number of skills related to attention, including complex scanning and visuomotor tracking and is considered to reflect the overall integrity of general brain functioning.

The TMT is a brief test, taking only 5 to 10 minutes to administer, and it has a wide age range of application (Spreen & Strauss 1998). It has, therefore, been used to evaluate a wide range of difficulties ranging from head injury to dementia and the detection of frontal lobe deficits.

Wisconsin Card Sorting Test (WCST)

The Wisconsin Card Sorting Test (WCST) (Grant & Berg 1993) is used primarily to assess abstract reasoning, concept generation and ideational perseveration. It is, therefore, considered to be sensitive to frontal lobe impairments and executive dysfunction. Basically, the patient is asked to sort cards according to rules and their performance is used to determine the ability to develop and maintain problem-solving strategies despite changing stimulus conditions.

The test can be given to 6.5 to 89 year olds and takes between 20 and 30 minutes to complete. It is available in a number of formats including an extended version and a computerized version.

Controlled Oral Word Association Test (COWAT)

The Controlled Oral Word Association Test (COWAT) consists of three timed naming trials in which the patient is asked to produce words beginning with the specific letters, F A and S but to exclude proper nouns, numbers and words with the same suffix. The test is useful in examining verbal knowledge and competency in abstract mental operations. It is, therefore, sensitive to a variety of CNS impairments and frontal lobe dysfunction in particular. It also benefits from being relatively brief to administer and can be given to a range of age groups (Spreen & Strauss 1998).

Cognitive Estimates Test (CET)

Based on the observation that questions that cannot be directly answered from general knowledge require novel reasoning and a comparison of the response with existing knowledge stores, the Cognitive Estimates Test (CET) (Shallice & Evans 1978) requires patients to estimate answers to questions such as: 'How fast do race horses gallop?', 'How heavy is a full pint of milk?', or 'How many camels are there in Holland?'

Being relatively brief to administer, the test is useful with adults and weighted heavily in favour of frontal lobe function. It can, therefore, be used as an indicator of frontal lobe disorder.

Judgement of Line Orientation (JLO)

Assessing visuospatial judgement, orientation and spatial perception, the Judgement of Line Orientation (JLO) (Benton et al 1994) is a simple and relatively brief test to administer. In short, the patient is asked to match a set of 30 test items of angled line stimuli with a card containing other, numbered angled lines.

Normative data for this test include age ranges from 16 to 74 years. A variation of this measure can also be seen as part of the RBANS visuospatial/constructional cognitive domain (see above).

Boston Diagnostic Aphasia Examination – third edition (BDAE-III)

Now in its third edition, the Boston Diagnostic Aphasia Examination (BDAE-III) (Goodglass et al 2000) is a test for aphasia. It contains a number of subtests examining fluency in naming, oral reading, reading comprehension, auditory comprehension, repetition, writing skills, and speech. The test can be used with adults and, in addition, a short form of the instrument allows for more rapid assessment. However, there is no time limit for test completion on the full assessment.

TESTS DESIGNED TO ASSESS PREMORBID FUNCTIONING

Estimates of an individual's level of general cognitive functioning prior to illness or injury allows us to estimate the degree of change or decline resulting from that injury or illness. One of the most widely used ways of estimating premorbid functioning is to measure reading ability since this is both highly correlated with general intelligence and more resistant to the changes observed with cerebral damage.

Wechsler Adult Test of Reading (WTAR)

The Wechsler Adult Test of Reading (WTAR) (Wechsler 2001) is designed to provide an estimation of premorbid intellectual functioning. Containing 50 words of increasingly complex, irregular pronunciation, the patient taking the test is asked to read each word aloud. Their correct or incorrect performance is noted on the record sheet and predicted estimates calculated.

The WTAR can be completed within about 10 minutes and be used to assess premorbid function levels in individuals ranging from 16 to 89 years. Results of the WTAR can be used to predict verbal, performance and full scale IQs on WAIS-III or the WASI (see above).

National Adult Reading Test (NART)

Like the WTAR (see above), the National Adult Reading Test (NART) and its more recent revised edition the NART-2 (Nelson & Wilson 1991), estimate premorbid intellectual ability through the assessment of reading skills. The NART-2 requires the patient to read 50 increasingly difficult and irregular words out loud. Their performance is noted and estimates of verbal, performance and full scale IQ calculated. These, in turn, can be interpreted against measures such as the WAIS-R, WASI-III, and WASI (see above).

The NART-2 is another brief test taking only some 10 minutes to complete and, again, can be used with a fairly wide age range of 16 to 70 years.

TESTS DESIGNED TO ASSESS PERSONALITY AND EMOTION

Emotional functioning and personality are also important factors to consider in neuropsychological assessment. Such instruments are able to assess the emotional impact of injuries and illness, evaluate adjustment, help to distinguish between normal and pathological responses, and assist in the differentiation of CNS impairment from the influence of emotional factors on test performance.

Hospital Anxiety and Depression Scale (HADS)

The Hospital Anxiety and Depression Scale (HADS) (Snaith & Zigmond 1994) is a brief self-report questionnaire which, despites its name, is a useful measure of levels of depression and generalized anxiety both inside and outside hospital settings. It allows for the identification of depression and anxiety symptomatology as well as offering a means to quantify these into categories of severity.

Beck Depression Inventory (BDI)

Available in a variety of forms, the latest version, the Beck Depression Inventory II (BDI II) (Beck et al 1996), is designed to assess depression in individuals aged 13 to 80 years. The test is, again, a brief self-report questionnaire that can also be administered verbally. It contains 21 items that are rated by the patient and it can be completed in around 5 minutes.

In addition, an even more rapid screening version of this test now exists that addresses the somatic and performance symptoms that were previously a problem for neuropsychologists. That is to say that previous versions of the test included a number of response choices that could be endorsed by patients suffering with the symptoms of neurological illness or trauma. This new version, then, was designed to reduce the number of false positive responses for depression in patients with known medical problems.

Beck Anxiety Inventory (BAI)

The Beck Anxiety Inventory (BAI) (Beck & Steer 1993) assesses the presence and severity of anxiety in adult and adolescent populations through the evaluation of the physiological and cognitive symptoms arising from the disturbance. Like the BDI (see above) this test is a self-report questionnaire, or it can be administered verbally, consisting of 21 items that are rated by the patient.

Minnesota Multiphasic Personality Inventory (MMPI-2)

The Minnesota Multiphasic Personality Inventory (MMPI-2) (Butcher et al 1989) is a large, self-administered personality inventory, and is used more frequently in the definition and diagnosis of psychological disorders than in neuropsychological settings. Consisting of 567 true or false questions, the MMPI-2 is used to identify psychopathology, assess the symptoms of social and personal maladjustment, identify treatment strategies, and support patient treatment and management decisions.

It contains a number of validity scales for assessing the patient's orientation to taking tests as well as a number of clinical scales including hypochondriasis, depression, conversion hysteria, psychopathic deviate, masculinity-femininity, paranoia, psychaesthenia, schizophrenia, hypomania and social introversion. In addition, it also contains a number of content and supplementary scales.

The test takes around 60 to 90 minutes to administer and can be used with individuals aged 18 years and older. The task of hand scoring this test and calculating the various subscales, content scores and excluding those items that have been shown to be endorsed by head injury, stroke and multiple sclerosis patients, etc., is time consuming, to say nothing of the experience and knowledge required to interpret the resultant patient profile. However, this has, to some degree, been helped by the evolution of computer software.

BRIEF SCREENING ASSESSMENTS

Very brief evaluations of general cognitive functioning are also available. These have the benefit of being very short in administration time, efficient in terms of assessment where more detailed tests are impractical, for example at the bedside or in cases where a more thorough assessment will not be tolerated by the patient, and, importantly, do not represent a discouragement to the patient. Such tests, however, suffer from not being very specific in their findings and, by their nature, have low cut-off scores in order to determine the presence of a cognitive problem, with the result that more subtle difficulties can be overlooked.

Mini-Mental Status Examination (MMSE)

Perhaps the most frequently encountered of these brief screening assessments is the Mini-Mental Status Examination (MMSE) (Folstein et al 1975). The MMSE is a brief measure of cognitive status in adults and is used to check for, estimate, and monitor levels of cognitive impairment. It takes only 5 minutes to complete and is frequently used in cases of neurodegenerative disorder, such as Alzheimer's disease, to monitor the efficacy of ongoing treatment.

Screening Test for the Luria-Nebraska Neuropsychological Battery (ST-LNNB)

This extremely short screening test, consisting of just 15 items from the LNNB, is used to predict probable performance on the full length battery. As such, the test is limited only to an indication of either 'normal' or 'abnormal' performance if the full test battery were to be administered. It cannot, therefore, be used to indicate deficit in a particular area.

Stroop Neuropsychological Screening Test (SNST)

The Stroop Neuropsychological Screening Test (SNST) (Trenerry et al 1989) is a brief procedure sensitive to difficulties in the ability to shift between conflicting verbal response modes, colour and words. As such, the SNST assesses speed of information processing, attentional skills, cognitive flexibility and resistance to distraction. In this form, it has been produced as a measure for use in the discrimination of brain-damaged individuals.

This very brief test can be administered in around 5 minutes and can be given to those aged 18 to 79 years.

Stroop Colour and Word Test (SCWT)

Like the SNST (see above), the Stroop Colour and Word Test (SCWT) (Golden 1978) is based on the observation that individuals are able to read words faster than they can identify colours, and like the SNST, it assesses cognitive flexibility, resistance to distraction and the ability to suppress competing verbal responses. This form of the test, however, is expanded, and again, this is to draw conclusions about possible cerebral dysfunction and psychopathology.

Again this instrument is very brief, taking around 5 minutes to complete, and can be applied across a number of age ranges from 15 to 90 years.

TEST OF MALINGERING

Finally, certain patients may demonstrate simulation or exaggeration of symptomatology; for example, patients involved in personal injury or criminal cases. Any battery of tests should, therefore, include at least some measurement of compliance and motivation that allows the test administrator to determine how much confidence it is possible to place in the results of the rest of their evaluation.

Examiners may be alerted to possible problems with dissimulation through the presentation of particular patients, the nature of the symptoms recounted by them or the over-endorsement of certain symptoms. For example, an examiner's index of suspicion might be raised if: a patient who complains of severe memory deficit appears to have no apparent problem in recalling detailed information from previous sessions; a patient demonstrates physical or cognitive symptoms that are extremely difficult to locate within what is known about normal function; or a patient endorses bizarre or outrageous symptoms.

In order to identify these potential problems, there are a number of procedures and test instruments available to assess this aspect of performance. Some are techniques that, on the surface look complex but are, in fact, relatively simple, for example the Rey Memory Test (RMT). Others rely on performance speed, such as the Dot Counting Test (DCT) or the superiority of some cognitive skills over others, for example the Test of Memory Malingering (TOMM). Others are computerized, such as the Victoria Symptom Validity Test (VST), while others represent profiles within other tests, for example the MMPI-2 (see above).

It must be kept in mind, however, that many of the symptoms presented by patients may at first appear strange, curious or singular. Nevertheless, as has been stated previously, this does not necessarily mean that such symptoms are not the signs of neuropsychological disturbance. It merely means that they appear remarkable before a full assessment has taken place. Dissimulation, lack of compliance and poor motivation, therefore, should be accepted as possibilities within each assessment. However, these factors should not be presumed to be present before all possible investigations to exclude their influence have been undertaken.

SUMMARY

This chapter, then, has offered a very brief explanation of the differences between neurological and neuropsychological testing. Moreover, it has provided an introduction to some of the more frequently encountered tests and assessments used by neuropsychologists and has given the reader some insight into the nature of these instruments.

We have examined a range of assessments designed to sample a range of cognitive functions, to assess single cognitive functions, to estimate premorbid ability, and those used to assess emotional and personality factors. Finally, we have given some thought to the issue of dissimulation and tests associated with this aspect of evaluation.

REFERENCES

Beck A T, Steer R A 1993 Beck anxiety inventory. Psychological Corporation, San Antonio

Beck A T, Steer R A, Brown G 1996 Beck depression inventory - II. Psychological Corporation, San Antonio

Benton A L, Sivan A B, des Hamsher K et al 1994 Contributions in neuropsychological assessment, 2nd edn. Oxford University Press, New York

Butcher J N, Dahlstrom W G, Graham J R et al 1989 MMPI-2: manual for administration and scoring. University of Minnesota Press, Minneapolis

Folstein M F, Folstein S E, McHugh P R 1975 Mini-mental state: a practical method for grading the cognitive state of patients for the clinician. Journal of Psychiatric Research 12:189–198

Golden C J 1978 Stroop color and word test. Stoelting, Chicago
Golden C J, Purisch A D, Hammeke T A 1985 Manual for the Luria-Nebraska neuropsychological battery: Forms I and II. Western Psychological Services, Los Angeles
Golding E 1989 Middlesex elderly assessment of mental state. Thames Valley Test Company, Cambridge
Goodglass H, Kaplan E, Barresi B 2000 Boston diagnostic aphasia examination, 3rd edn. Lee & Febiger, Philadelphia
Grant D A, Berg E A 1993 Wisconsin card sort test. Psychological Assessment Resources, Odessa
Gronwall D M A 1977 Paced auditory serial-addition task: a measure of recovery from concussion. Perceptual and Motor Skills 44:367–373
Leach L, Kaplan E, Rewlilak D et al 2000 Kaplan baycrest neurocognitive assessment. Psychological Corporation, San Antonio
Mattis S, Jurica P J, Leitten C 2002 Dementia rating scale – 2. Psychological Corporation, San Antonio
Nelson H E, Wilson J 1991 National adult reading test, 2nd edn. Nfer-Nelson, London
Randolph C 1998 Repeatable battery for the assessment of neuropsychological status. Psychological Corporation, San Antonio
Reitan R M, Wolfson D 1993 The Halstean-Reitan neuropsychological test battery: theory and clinical interpretation. Neuropsychological Press, Tucson
Robertson I H, Ward T, Ridgeway V et al 1994 Test of everyday attention. Thames Valley Test Company; Cambridge
Saxton J, McGonigle K L, Swihart A A, et al 1993 Severe impairment battery. Thames Valley Test Company, Cambridge
Shallice T, Evans M E 1978 The involvement of the frontal lobes in cognitive estimation. Cortex 14:294–303
Snaith R P, Zigmond A S 1994 Hospital anxiety and depression scale. Nfer-Nelson, London
Spreen O, Strauss E 1998 Compendium of neuropsychological tests: administration, norms, and commentary, 2nd edn. Oxford University Press, New York
Trenerry M R, Crosson B, DeBoe J et al 1989 The Stroop neuropsychological screening test. Psychological Assessment Resources, Odessa
Wechsler D 2003 Wechsler memory scale third edition abbreviated. Psychological Corporation, San Antonio
Wechsler D 2001 Wechsler test of adult reading. Psychological Corporation, San Antonio
Wechsler D 1999 Manual for the Wechsler abbreviated scale of intelligence. Psychological Corporation, San Antonio
Wechsler D 1997a Administration and scoring manual for the Wechsler adult intelligence scale - third edition. Psychological Corporation, San Antonio
Wechsler D 1997b Administration and scoring manual for the Wechsler memory scale - third edition. Psychological Corporation, San Antonio
Wilson B A, Cockburn J, Baddeley A 2003 The Rivermead behavioural memory test - 2nd edition. Thames Valley Test Company, Cambridge

FURTHER READING

Evans J E, Wilson B A, Emslie H 1996 Selecting, administering and interpreting cognitive tests. Thames Valley Test Company, Bury St. Edmunds.
Hebben N, Milberg W 2002 Essentials of neuropsychological assessment. Wiley, New York
Spreen O, Strauss E 1998 Compendium of neuropsychological tests: administration, norms, and commentary, 2nd edn. Oxford University Press, New YorkI

Initial assessment

11

OVERVIEW

So far, we have looked at the structure of the nervous system, methods of investigation, behavioural neuroanatomy, psychological and emotional processes, the more frequently encountered neurological disorders, some of the more unusual signs and symptoms, recovery mechanisms, and introduced formal neuropsychological testing. In order to put this new learning into perspective and make practical use of this knowledge, we will now turn our attention to the basic assessment techniques that can be employed to help provide insight into the neuropsychological impairments experienced by patients.

Before doing so, however, it must be stressed that the contents of this chapter are not intended to provide a substitute for professional neuropsychological assessment. Nor is it proposed that the procedures listed below offer a replacement for specialist training. Some patients will present with complex problems and their referral is essential for satisfactory interpretation. Still others will present with confusing and extremely difficult complaints, emphasizing the need for careful and informed quantification, further underscoring the previously stated observation that what you see is not always what you get.

However, with these provisos in mind, it has been my experience that there is often some apprehension in the appraisal of neuropsychological problems that could be addressed through an adequate grounding in evaluation practices. Such an undertaking, I believe, would both afford the nurse or allied health professional more confidence in their observations and make for a more efficient and effective use of the services available.

To this end, therefore, we will examine the importance of the history, medical record and pathogenesis of a condition. We will then discuss what can be done by those with more regular exposure to the patient to initially evaluate suspected impairment before deciding that a referral for further assessment and treatment is needed.

BACKGROUND TO ASSESSMENT

When assessing for central nervous system (CNS) involvement it is important to remember that the behavioural manifestations of such involvement can be very varied. Some patients with neurological or neuropsychological impairments may exhibit specific and localizable signs such as aphasia. In other cases, however, there may appear to be widespread impairments such as a generalized deficit in almost all cognitive abilities. Even the presenting deficits themselves may range from the very subtle to the very severe and may be obscured or amplified by additional emotional components.

The practical implication of such variation is that there is no single, brief, fixed approach to screening for neuropsychological impairment that can assess the broad range of abilities expressed. Any such approach would, therefore, only be likely to assess a very narrow range of the patient's abilities and fail to produce an adequate profile of deficits if such problems were to fall outside the range of skills tested. The probable outcome of such a procedure, then, would be a high number of false negative observations.

As explained in Chapter 10, formalized, brief, screening assessment tools do exist. The Mini-Mental Status Test (MMSE) is a relatively unsophisticated instrument that samples a narrow band of cognitive skills. As such, it benefits from being short, portable, and easy to administer, score and interpret. It has, therefore, been used to great effect to screen for gross cognitive difficulties in a range of populations. However, the very qualities that make the MMSE so useful also make it a rather blunt instrument that cannot isolate some of the more subtle difficulties encountered.

An alternative strategy, then, that seeks to reduce the influence of these problems is to perform an expanded and more fluid assessment, which is tailored to the needs of the patient and customized to evaluate a wider range of abilities. Such an assessment, although longer than the MMSE, might still be relatively quick and simple to administer but sample a wider array of cognitive skills. To this end, then, a combination of the tasks provided below might fulfil such criteria.

THE HISTORY AND MEDICAL RECORD

Before more formally assessing the patient, however, it may be useful to get some understanding of the background to their presentation and the evolution of their problems. What is the diagnosis? Are there comorbid conditions present that might influence neuropsychological presentation?

At this stage, then, an interrogation of the medical record with regard to significant historical features may prove constructive, for the answers to many questions surrounding current presentation may lie in past events, illnesses or occupation, etc. Thus, the importance of understanding the patient's history cannot be over emphasized.

In terms of the family history it may be useful to determine if there are any known conditions that could influence the current situation. For example, are there any conditions with a known or suspected genetic component? Is there a family history of medical problems such as heart disease or stroke? Is there any evidence of learning disability, premature deaths or atypical behaviour in the family?

Although not often available, prenatal and early personal history details can provide useful information. For example, is it possible that the patient was exposed to toxic agents such as pesticides, solvents, drugs, or alcohol while in utero? Were there any birth complications? Were there any developmental delays?

Details of the patient's occupational history can also prove enlightening. For instance, a patient's occupational history can help to establish estimates of the premorbid level of functioning. Occupational details might also help to suggest avenues for further investigation. For example, a farm worker may have been occupationally exposed to organophosphates. Furthermore, many occupations will over-develop certain cognitive skills and, therefore, might have an impact on assessment. For example, an accountant may have well-developed arithmetic skills.

The patient's medical history is also an important source of information and a review of the patient's medical notes can often help to determine if current symptoms can be accounted for based on a medical complaint. For example, does the patient have a history of epilepsy that could be associated with transient memory difficulties; or could the medication regimen produce cognitive side-effects?

Most importantly, careful observations of the patient's current status and evolution of their cognitive symptoms can provide a wealth of data that might contribute to current presentation. Each symptom should, therefore, be assessed in the light of its onset, frequency, duration, intensity and qualities, over time.

For example, attentional problems that have produced a mild difficulty with concentration may have coincided with a relatively mild closed head injury 2 months prior to assessment and which now shows signs of resolution. Alternatively, a patient demonstrating signs of agitation may habitually drink litres of caffeine-rich soft drinks per day and be demonstrating signs of a substance-induced problem rather than symptoms of a psychopathological process.

Next, it may be prudent to examine the medical record and look particularly at any laboratory results and/or neurological investigations. Although care is needed in the interpretation of such results, one might ask the questions: are there any suspect haematological, biochemical, or microbiological results? Has an electroencephalography (EEG), computed tomography (CT), magnetic resonance imaging (MRI) or other scan been performed? If so what were the results?

Remember that CT scans, despite their inherent technological advantages, can still be insensitive to certain conditions. For example, CT can overlook subcortical white matter changes and it can miss subtle alterations in the CNS tissues caused by traumatic brain injury.

MRI scans are, generally, more sensitive than CT but are still not perfect. For example, sometimes MRI can overestimate CNS involvement in some conditions. Some types of MRI can overrate periventricular white matter involvement. Thus, sufferers of chronic migraine can sometimes demonstrate white matter lesions, which, to the untrained eye, can mimic the changes associated with multiple sclerosis.

Medications are also useful to consider as there are many drugs that can influence neuropsychological performance as a side-effect. For example:

some drugs given in cases of Parkinson's disease can produce hallucinations, hypomania, and/or paranoia; some anticonvulsants can produce ataxia, dysarthria or confusion; diuretics can produce tinnitus; while antiarrythmics are able to generate hallucinations and depression.

PHYSICAL EXAMINATION

While physical examination is best left to those with more experience and training in the subtleties of presentation, it is often helpful to have at least some knowledge of the practicalities of such observations.

To begin with, most physical assessments of the CNS begin with an evaluation of the cranial nerves. The cranial nerves may each be individually tested by means of the presentation of stimuli or by the observation of the action or inaction associated with a particular nerve. Below are just a few examples of the testing procedures.

The first cranial nerve, the olfactory nerve, may be tested by the application of specific odours to each nostril and requesting the patient to identify them. Such procedures may not, at first, appear to have a practical application. However, it should be recalled that olfactory hallucinations often occur with temporal lobe epilepsy and that olfactory acuity can often be lowered in cases of dementia.

Similarly, the second cranial nerve, the optic nerve, can be examined in a variety of ways. Visual acuity is measured by way of Snellen charts. The extent of the peripheral visual fields, on the other hand, can be assessed by asking the patient to indicate when they observe a target object moved from the outer to the inner portion of each quadrant of the visual field of each eye.

Simultaneous visual stimulation may be assessed by asking the patient to fix their gaze on the examiner's eyes or nose. The patient is then asked to identify finger movements made by the examiner in the extremes of their upper and lower visual fields. First, single movements are attempted and then the patient is asked to identify simultaneous movement. If the patient is able to perceive single movements but not simultaneous movements, this could indicate contralateral dysfunction in the visual system and the possible presence of simultagnosia.

The third, fourth and sixth cranial nerves, the oculomotor, trochlear and abducens, respectively, control ocular motility and the pupil. The direct reaction of the pupil to light is tested by way of a pen torch shone into the eye. An indirect pupil reflex can also be observed if a light is again shone into one eye but the reaction of the other pupil is observed. This is known as the consensual reflex. The third and fourth nerves may be tested by asking the patient to track target objects up and down with their eyes. The sixth nerve is assessed by asking the patient to visually track objects left and right.

The fifth cranial nerve, the trigeminal nerve, supplies portions of the face, and is divided into both motor and sensory portions. Sensation may be assessed by the application of cotton or a pin in a light touch to the upper and lower jaw and the forehead. The motor division of the nerve may be assessed through the observation of possible deviations in the movement of the mouth on opening.

The seventh cranial nerve or facial nerve again supplies portions of the face and is involved in taste sensation. Motor action of the seventh nerve can be observed by assessing facial movement, both in conversation and to command, while looking for evidence of asymmetry in facial movement. Taste sensations are, however, more difficult to evaluate. Nevertheless, sweet, sour and salt sensations can be elicited through the application of appropriate stimuli to specific portions of the tongue.

The eighth cranial nerve, the acoustic or vestibulocochlear nerve, is involved in hearing. Deafness and tinnitus can obviously suggest the involvement of the acoustic nerve. However, complaints of vertigo may also be associated with dysfunction related to the vestibular system. Acuity is assessed by asking the patient to cover one ear while the examiner whispers into the other. Alternatively, the examiner may lightly rub their fingers together or ask the patient if they can hear a wristwatch near their ear. Tuning forks may also be used to assess the difference between sound carried through the air and sound conducted through the bones of the skull (Rinne's and Weber's tests).

The ninth, tenth and twelfth cranial nerves, the glossopharyngeal, vagus and hypoglossal nerves, respectively, are involved with brain stem functions. Assessment involves the evaluation of tongue movements in the mouth, the movement of the uvula, the quality of speech, swallowing and the gag reflex.

Finally, the eleventh cranial nerve, the accessory nerve, is involved in motor function. It may be assessed by asking the patient to perform movements such as shrugging the shoulders or turning the head.

Evaluation of the cranial nerves is followed by examination of the motor system, looking at strength, coordination and tone. Deep tendon reflexes are tested, assessing the integrity of the reflex arcs underlying them, and observations are made with regard to the presence of fasiculations, tremor, spasticity, rigidity, weakness or paralysis.

Tests in this area are many and varied. However, a few examples of the more common assessments may serve to illustrate the type and nature of these evaluations. For instance, abnormalities in the organization or amplitude of movement of the hands with rapidly alternating movement might suggest dysdiadochokinesia and possibly the presence of cerebellar dysfunction; heel to toe or tandem walking, both backward and forward, might reveal difficulties with balance and coordination; postural arm drift while the patient has their eyes closed and their arms extended horizontally might suggest dysfunction in the cerebral hemisphere contralateral to the drift.

Finally, sensory system examination assesses a number of symptoms such as paraesthesia, anaesthesia, pain, and reduced or lost sensation through the perception of temperature, pain, light touch, vibration sense and two-point discrimination. In addition, patients are asked frequently to assess the weight, size, shape and texture of objects.

In addition to these more fundamental examinations, a number of other miscellaneous physical signs may also be elicited during the course of assessment. Again, these are numerous and varied. However, several of them may be useful to describe here as they have a direct bearing on the next section concerning higher function assessment. Amongst these are the Babinski reflex and Hoover's sign and the more primitive grasping, pout, suckling, glabbellar tap, and palmomental reflexes, all of which could suggest the involvement of the frontal lobes.

The grasp reflex may be elicited by a stroke of the palm of the hand. A positive response consists of an involuntary grasping on the part of the patient. Such a sign is almost always pathological in younger patients, but may be observed normally in the elderly.

Pouting reflexes may be elicited by asking the patient to close their eyes and then stimulating the mid-point of the lips with a tap. A positive response consists of a projection or pouting of the lips towards the stimulus. A suckling reflex, on the other hand, involves the stimulation of the angle of the mouth resulting in a suckling action. Again, such a sign observed in younger patients could suggest pathology but may be normal for elderly patients.

The glabellar tap reflex may be obtained by tapping in the mid-line between the eyebrows. Normally, a blink in response after the first three or four taps will be inhibited. However, a failure to inhibit this response after five or more taps is considered positive.

The palmomental reflex, also known as the palm-chin reflex (or Radovici's sign) may be elicited by pressure on the thenar eminence (the mound of the palm at the base of the thumb) in the palm. A positive response results in the contraction of the mentalis muscle in the chin.

The Babinski reflex is elicited by stimulation of the sole of the foot. Dorsiflection of the big toe due to this stimulation of the sole is of little localizing significance but does suggest CNS involvement.

Finally, and in contrast to the above reflexes, Hoover's sign is observed in some patients who may not be putting forth full voluntary effort on motor testing; that is, possibly not fully complying with the examination. In this case the patient is supine. The examiner's hands are placed underneath each of the patient's heels and the patient is then asked to raise each leg individually. Downward pressure on the hand underneath the heel of the opposite leg should be felt if voluntary effort is intact or unless genuine paralysis is present.

OBSERVATIONS BEFORE AND DURING TESTING

Before going on to assess cognitive functioning it is essential to have some idea of the patient's motivational and emotional state. If individuals taking the test do not cooperate with the evaluation because of extreme depression or anxiety, or if they are suffering from an obvious problem that will influence test performance, such as aphasia, the resulting impact on test performance could produce false positive results or distort outcomes sufficiently to make the process all but useless. It is vital, then, to have some understanding of the patient's level of motivation and emotional state prior to testing.

In addition, a note of behaviour should be kept during testing. Do patients maintain an adequate level of alertness during the procedure? Are they easily fatigued? Can they maintain their attention to the test tasks? Does extraneous environmental noise distract them? Are their behavioural responses appropriate during the procedure? These and other questions regarding an individual's test-taking behaviour should be kept in mind throughout the process and significant observations noted, as such observations can both serve to qualify test results and lend weight to the test findings.

For example, patients who are extremely depressed might demonstrate poor results on testing, not because they are necessarily impaired, which they might well be, but because their emotional state prevented an accurate assessment. Or, a patient who is easily fatigued might demonstrate a tailing off of performance towards the end of a testing procedure. The impact on their test result, therefore, could suggest problems with later items in the testing process. More likely, however, is the influence of reduced arousal on test performance and, thus, a different interpretation of their test outcomes.

These considerations, on the surface, appear to increase the complexity of the testing procedure and seem to add yet another tier of observational data to what may already be an intricate process. However, when one considers these various factors it is clear that many of them are components of behaviour that we observe all of the time and, for the most part, hide in plain sight.

In short, we are commonly aware of many of these aspects of behaviour but, generally, do not specifically note them or make efforts to record them formally, often because, although important, they have little bearing on our usual practices. To illustrate, depression will likely have little effect on the efficacy of an intra-muscular injection. However, in terms of basic cognitive testing, because of the importance of such observations and the effect that many of these factors can have, it is prudent to be aware of these overt behaviours and to document any significant impact these could have on test procedures.

BASIC COGNITIVE ASSESSMENT

The following basic assessment strategies are an expansion of those found on the MMSE and sample a wider range of cognitive skills. Unlike the MMSE, procedures detailed here offer only a limited amount of scoring, providing no specific cut-off point for what may be categories such as 'normal' or 'abnormal'. However, while not offering that reassuringly simple dichotomy of categorization, these measures do afford the examiner a greater insight into the neuropsychological functioning and some of the impairments encountered.

Orientation

Orientation questions access the patient's current knowledge base with regard to what most of us refer to as time, place and person. In so doing, this measure is gauging the examinee's declarative memory, their fund of personally relevant information and their estimation of the passage of time. A format for such enquiries might be:

- Time
  - Time of day
  - Season
  - Day
  - Date
  - Month
  - Year
- Place
  - Building
  - Town
  - County
  - Country
- Person
  - Name
  - Age
  - Date of birth

Interpretation of the responses to such questions can obviously indicate difficulties with orientation. It should be remembered, however, that errors can occur on this measure that do not necessarily indicate difficulties. To illustrate, mistakes within the days and dates do not inevitably mean a high level of disorientation if there is some degree of consistency. For example, providing a date within 2 days of the actual date or providing a day of the week within 1 day of the actual day may not provide evidence of disorientation: with in-patient settings, hospital environments may not be conducive to the accurate maintenance of such information.

Attention

Attentional measures focus on the patient's ability to concentrate on a task and manipulate information in working memory. Such brief tests, then, assess the ability to select and sustain cognitive effort and, to some degree, the ability to monitor ongoing performance.

A number of such brief tests, each of which can be used in isolation, can be given if the patient fails on other tasks, or can be administered in addition to single measures to provide ever more complex and demanding tasks.

One might, therefore, ask the examinee to recite the months of the year or the days of the week backwards. This has the value of using something that is familiar but avoids a simple repetition of information that may have become over-learned or habitual. Similarly, the examinee might be asked to spell a familiar word backwards, for example, 'world' as 'dlrow'.

Another more intensive technique is to ask an examinee to repeat increasingly complex strings of single digits presented orally. In this instance, the task is divided into two trials: forwards and backwards. The examiner first reads out a list of single digits at a rate of one per second in the forwards trial. Starting with simple strings and moving to increasingly longer strings of numbers, the examinee is asked to repeat each string. The examiner records either a pass or a fail on the examinee's part and moves onto the next string, and so on. A failure on two strings of equal length is the point at which the trial is discontinued. An example of digit span strings is shown in Box 11.1.

Box 11.1 Example of digit span strings

Forwards string	*Backwards string*
5-8-2	3-9
3-7-2	6-2
3-7-2-5	5-6-9
9-2-6-4	6-4-3
4-2-7-3-1	9-2-6-4
8-4-6-1-9	1-7-5-3
9-3-7-4-6-1	3-9-2-4
2-8-1-3-9-7	4-1-7-9
4-7-5-3-8-6-2	2-7-3-6-8
1-4-9-3-7-4-5	7-5-8-3-6

Next the examinee is asked to repeat the process for the backwards trial of the test, except that this time, on each occasion that they are asked to repeat a string, they must reverse it. For example, if the string of numbers is 1-2-3, the examinee must respond with 3-2-1, and so on.

A normal digit span on the forwards trial of the test is six numbers, plus or minus one. On the backwards trial, a more complex task, normal responses are usually five numbers plus or minus one. In addition, a useful rule of thumb suggests that all other factors being taken into account, a digit span of three or less on the backwards trial can indicate cerebral pathology.

A more complex and potentially more intimidating task to measure attentional skills is to ask the patient to serially subtract 7, starting with 100. That is to say, the examinee must subtract 7 from 100, which leaves 93; they must then subtract 7 from this answer, leaving 86, and so on. Obviously, this is a useful measure of attention skills, working memory and, to some degree, calculation. However, this measure can, on the surface, appear to be too much, even for those of us with fairly well-developed mathematical skills. It is also important to keep in mind that the important factor here is a consistent ability to maintain a correct response in subtraction rather than highlighting single instances of errors. For example, a patient may incorrectly subtract 7 from 86 but, thereafter, preserve the integrity of their calculations.

Memory

As we have already observed in previous chapters, memory functioning relies on a number of cognitive systems and is supported by the intact functioning of a number of brain structures. Furthermore, there are various types of memory, for example explicit and implicit, and short-term and long-term that can demonstrate differing types of deficit.

Rapid and specific testing of all of the facets of memory functioning is, therefore, beyond the scope of a brief assessment. It is, however, possible to examine gross functioning through assessment on simple procedures. This can provide information on verbal memory functioning as well as, to a lesser degree, non-verbal or visual memory functioning in both anterograde and retrograde modalities.

In terms of anterograde functioning, one might ask the patient to repeat a list of items three times and then recall it. For example, the examinee is told that they will be asked to immediately recall the words 'apple', 'book' and 'tree' after three repetitions, or they may be asked to identify and recall three simple items presented visually, such as 'pen', 'watch', and 'key'. Delayed recall for visual or verbal information is then tested some 5 minutes later by asking the patient to recall the items memorized.

A slightly more complex but similar verbal task is to have the patient memorize a simple address, for example:

Paul Richards
31 High Street
Exeter
Devon

The address, comprising seven items, is repeated three times in order to check that it has been attended to and registered correctly. After each repetition a note of the number of items correctly recalled is made. Following a delay of 5 minutes, the patient is then asked to recall the address and a note is again made of the correct or incorrect recall for the seven items provided.

A more detailed assessment of visual memory functioning is extremely difficult in situations that demand a relatively unsophisticated test format. However, some information can be gathered through observation of patients and their ability to remember routes in familiar environments, recollect faces, or recall the details of visually presented images. Another very simple and blunt means of testing visual memory might be to use the intersecting polygon and other visual copy tasks used later on under Visuoconstructional Functioning.

More distant memories present a more difficult area of enquiry as the nature of these is influenced by exposure limitations, subjective personal interpretations, individual preferences, and so on. Nevertheless, remote memory can be assessed through an appreciation of the patient's ability to recall autobiographical data and to recollect the details of events.

Accessing autobiographical recall can, however, be tricky, for the simple reason that most of us will have little or no knowledge of the patient's previous life experiences and, therefore, no yardstick for measurement. Without depending on more formal assessment techniques, the best that can be hoped for is an impression of functional integrity. Therefore, in conversations with patients, their ability to discuss events in their earlier lives, such as school attendance, marriages or jobs, might form the basis of our opinions.

With regard to an appreciation of the patient's recall of factual information surrounding prominent events, we must be aware of the personal and cultural factors that can influence these; for example someone who does not support the royal family is unlikely to recall the marriage of the Prince of Wales to Diana Spencer; and a person not interested in sports is unlikely to recall who won the world cup in 1966.

Assessment in this area, then, will necessarily mean some understanding of patients' likes and dislikes, their personal preferences and, to some degree, their subjective predilections. Nevertheless, it is possible, with these qualifications in mind, to gain some insight into functioning, since a great many events unconnected with our personal preferences will have come to our attention.

One might, therefore, ask the examinee to recall who the prime minister is, to recount the name of the previous prime minister or provide the name of the president of the United States. Similarly, the examinee may be asked to recount details regarding the fall of the Berlin Wall, the decline of communism in Russia, the events surrounding the invasion of Iraq, or their recollections of the September 11th terrorist attack on the World Trade Centre.

Speech and language

Assessment of speech and language functions will endeavour to evaluate the quality of speech, comprehension, repetition, naming skills, reading skills and writing skills. Such testing allows us to gain some insight into possible aphasic problems, paraphasic intrusions, articulation and fluency difficulties, syntactic errors, prosodic dysfunctions, word-finding deficits, and understanding.

Being aware that, like memory functioning, speech and language patterns are highly individual, we can begin by assessing the patient's spontaneous speech, that which is not elicited by specific tests. The overall quality of such spontaneous speech can be graded according to the level of articulation, the presence of dysarthria and dysphonia, the complexity of expressions, the degree of fluency observed in linguistic operations, the syntax or grammar used, the prosodic or melodic qualities of utterances and the presence of significant word-finding difficulties and paraphasic errors.

More formal testing of a patient's speech and language abilities can also be achieved through the administration of a number of relatively simple tests. These involve a more active evaluation of individual processes and require patients to provide fairly fixed responses to requests.

Naming skills can be affected by a number of cerebral pathologies. Here patients are assessed by asking them to name objects such as a pen or a watch. The degree of difficulty observed with such a task increases with the decreasing familiarity of an object. To illustrate, 'pen' and 'watch' are what are known as high frequency words; that is to say, we encounter them with fairly high frequency. However, 'syringe' and 'stethoscope' are lower frequency words because we encounter them with less frequency.

Similarly, comprehension skills can be affected in an increasingly complex manner. To assess the possible level of comprehension difficulty, it is usual to start with simpler single word understanding and increase the level of complexity to simple and then more complex sentences.

A patient, therefore, may be asked to point to single objects within the room. Again, lower and higher frequency objects will tend to produce similar patterns to the naming task. Next, the patient may be asked to comprehend the syntactic meaning of sentences and asked to carry out simple actions; for example, the patient may be asked to place the pen on the chair or touch the cup to the paper.

The level of complexity may then be increased by the examiner in order to assess the impact of less concrete concepts on comprehension. For example, the patient may be asked to pick out an object used to record the passage of time or to point to the object used for writing. Alternatively, the patient may be asked what the hard outer casing of animals such as snails is called.

Lastly, the patient may be asked to complete a more complex command. Frequently, the patient is asked:

- 'Take this piece of paper in your right hand, fold it in half and put it on the floor.'

Repetition skills can be affected by certain types of aphasia; and repetition skills tests can also reveal articulatory problems despite intact language functioning. Problems may be elicited by asking the patient to repeat single words, followed by sentences or phrases such as:

- 'No ifs, ands or buts.'
- 'British constitution.'
- 'Baby hippopotamus.'
- 'The guard whistled and the train began to move.'

Writing skills, like spoken language skills, may be assessed by both observations of spontaneous behaviour and more formal testing strategies in order to examine the possible presence of dysgraphia. First, it is possible to sample patients' writing skills through observation of functioning when they are asked to freely compose sentences and passages on subjects of their own choosing. Secondly, patients can be asked to write down a sentence that is dictated.

By using such methods, evidence of a number of problems can be found. It should be remembered, however, that the results of these tasks may need to be compared to performance within other areas of assessment in order to exclude the influence of other factors. For example, a comparison of dictated writing tasks with oral comprehension results can indicate that it is understanding of the spoken word that is impaired rather than writing skills. Similarly, a comparison to motor functioning performance can also help to exclude praxis problems as another possible source of discrepancy.

Simple reading skills can be assessed by asking the patient to read aloud simple lists of words, followed by sentences, followed by a whole passage. Reading skills are, of course, linked with educational background and must also be considered first in order to rule out a problem in understanding.

The ability to comprehend what one is being asked to read is also important. Assessment prior to a more formalized or intensive evaluation serves to both exclude the influence of a comprehension problem and help to highlight otherwise overlooked problems such as reduced visual acuity. Testing is achieved by writing down a simple command and asking the patient to perform it. For example:

- 'Close your eyes.'
- 'Raise your hands.'
- 'Nod your head if you are male/female.'

Alternatively, if a more complex assessment of reading comprehension is required, then the patient can be asked to read a passage from a book, newspaper or magazine and then discuss it with the examiner.

Calculation

Assessing numerical skills is useful in terms of primary arithmetic functioning. It is, however, also a useful marker of further language problems, such as reading and comprehension of numbers, as well as being an indicator of attentional skills. A distinction is made here between a difficulty with numbers per se, acalculia, and difficulty with mathematical computation, anarithmetria. Testing in this area, then, is hierarchical, moving from simple number reading and writing to more complex oral and written arithmetic.

Thus, the examinee is first asked to read numbers aloud from a written list, such as 2, 13, 18, 108, and 1032. Next the examinee is asked to write down numbers presented orally, such as 3, 7, 9, 10, 256, and 1024. The examinee may then be asked to copy numbers and to point to numbers presented to them orally. Such simple procedures allow the examiner to assess the linguistic components of numerical skill and exclude factors such as alexia for numbers and agraphia for numbers.

The examinee is then asked to complete a number of increasingly difficult oral and written mathematical problems. It is at this stage that attentional functioning difficulties may also be observed. Oral arithmetic, therefore, might include items such as:

- 3 + 4 (7)
- 12 + 7 (19)
- 17 + 26 (43)
- 12 – 7 (5)
- 35 – 8 (27)
- 63 – 17 (46)

Written arithmetic, using a piece of paper to both write down the problem and to record the steps used in working the problem out, will help to both provide evidence of spatial problems and incorrect number alignment, and help to support memory functions. Problems in this area may, therefore, be a little more complex and might include items such as:

- 8 + 2 (10)
- 14 + 12 (26)
- 64 + 27 (91)
- 132 + 256 (388)
- 17 – 5 (12)
- 38 – 16 (22)
- 101 – 19 (82)

- 3 × 2 (6)
- 7 × 6 (42)
- 13 × 14 (182)
- 112 × 7 (784)
- 12 ÷ 2 (6)
- 28 ÷ 7 (4)
- 132 ÷ 6 (22)

Executive function

As previously described in Chapter 3 the executive functions encompass a broad set of cognitive abilities necessary for independent functioning. However, the nature of these abilities makes them extremely difficult to measure directly. Without recourse to more sophisticated techniques, then, the assessment of executive functioning therefore involves the testing of some skills associated with the intact functioning of the frontal lobes.

In the absence of aphasic problems, verbal fluency abilities have long been associated with the integrity of frontal lobe functioning. A means of testing such skills requires the patient to generate words beginning with specific letters of the alphabet. The patient is given 60 seconds to generate words in each category and is instructed that no proper nouns can be used (words that would be capitalized in use, such as Birmingham or Brian); that they cannot repeat words; and that they cannot use words with the same prefix, such as 'sun', 'sunshine', 'sunbath' and 'sunbeam'.

The most frequently used letters are F, A and S and the patient's total score for all words across each category is assessed. Performance depends on age and, again, educational background. These factors should, therefore, be considered along with the results of the test. Nevertheless, generally speaking, patients should not perseverate and a total correct word generation of thirty or less is considered abnormal. This cut-off point is, of course, lowered for elderly patients and those cases where a low educational attainment is suspected. In these cases a total score of twenty five correct words in total is considered abnormal.

The ability to form concepts and perform abstract interpretations has also been associated with frontal lobe functioning and a variety of methods to examine these abilities have been defined in order to gain some insight into levels of functioning. One method involves the interpretation of proverbs, another, the relationship between pairs of items.

Proverb interpretation requires the patient to provide an explanation of maxims. In cases where frontal lobe functioning is intact it is usual to receive an analogous or abstract interpretation. However, in cases where frontal lobe dysfunction occurs a more concrete interpretation is usually given. For example, in response to 'Strike while the iron is hot', instead of providing the answer 'Do things while the opportunity exists', the patient with frontal lobe damage may reply 'Hit the metal while it is still warm'.

Naturally, such interpretations are highly dependant on educational and cultural background and it is extremely important to assess these factors before interpreting responses. With these qualifications in mind, then, a few examples of these sayings might include:

- 'Still waters run deep.'
- 'One swallow does not a summer make.'
- 'Strike while the iron is hot.'

The patient's ability to discern the conceptual relationship between items can also be explored by asking them what is similar with regard to increasingly abstract pairs of items. For example, an early item such as 'What is similar about an apple and orange?' would elicit the response 'They're both fruit'. Later items, however, are more abstract and can therefore elicit more concrete responses. For example, 'What is similar about a table and chair?' might elicit the response 'You can sit on both of them' rather than 'They're both items of furniture'.

Again, more concrete responding is anticipated with frontal lobe involvement. However, educational history again plays a substantial role and must be taken into account when assessing this ability. Examples of these pairings, arranged in a more concrete to abstract format, include:

- Apple and orange (fruit)
- Dog and lion (animals)
- Coat and suit (clothing)
- Table and chair (furniture)
- Poem and statue (works of art)
- Praise and punishment (means of modifying behaviour).

Another ability mediated by the frontal lobes is the capacity to inhibit responses and sequence action. The subtle range of difficulties observed in this area precludes all but the most simple of motor testing. Nevertheless, some useful information can be gathered by evaluation of gross motor functioning in the absence of other motor dysfunctions such as paresis.

First, in order to evaluate the patient's ability to inhibit motor responses a tapping test can be performed. Here, the examiner, having first checked that the patient's hearing is adequate to the task, uses a pen, pencil or similar implement to tap on a hard surface such as a table-top. The patient is instructed to either tap the table-top twice, if they hear only one tap from the examiner, or tap the table-top once if they hear two taps from the examiner. Over a sequence of trials the examiner notes the responses of the patient and their ability to perform correctly.

Sequencing motor action is another problem that patients with frontal lobe damage can often exhibit. In order to test this, the patient is asked to make rapidly alternating movements with the hands. To illustrate, the examiner demonstrates by extending the fingers on one hand while clenching the fingers of the other (Fig. 11.1). This hand position is then reversed so that the fingers on the clenched hand are extended and the fingers on the extended hand are clenched into a fist. After demonstrating this movement, the patient is asked to repeat the movement as fast as they are able eight times.

The examiner may then observe a very slow but accurate performance, a loss of sequencing, a production of the same movement in both hands, or a

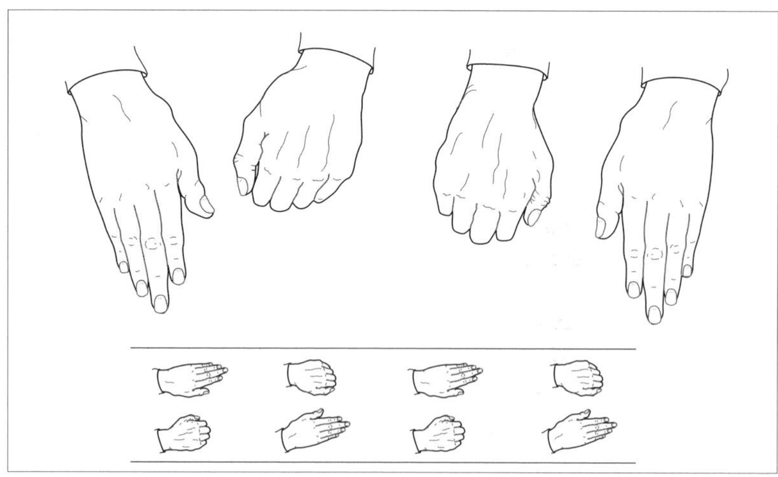

Fig. 11.1 The hand movements of alternating motor functioning.

complete inability to perform the task. Problems with this task can suggest problems with frontal lobe functioning. However, it should also be kept in mind that such alternating movement problems are not limited to dysfunction associated with the frontal lobe and can also be observed in disorders affecting other brain structures.

Praxis

Assessment of praxis tests for the presence of ideomotor apraxia, a difficulty with the ability to perform skilful or purposeful movements to command. Another form known as ideational apraxia, a difficulty in the use of objects secondary to problems with object identification or problems with the conceptualization of object use is, obviously, more difficult to assess, and therefore not easily accessible.

In this area, the examinee is asked to perform a series of transitive and intransitive facial and limb movements. That is to say that the patient is requested to perform intransitive actions that may be interpreted as restricted to gesturing, such as waving or beckoning; or transitive actions that involve the use of objects, such as using scissors or combing the hair.

Items in this category of tests are also broken down into limb and facial performance tasks indicating limb apraxia or buccofacial apraxia. The patient is first asked to show the examiner how they would:

- *Intransitive limb movements*
  - Wave goodbye
  - Motion 'come here'
  - Thumb or hitch a ride
  - Signal someone to 'stop'
  - Perform a salute

- *Transitive limb movements*
  - Use scissors
  - Brush teeth
  - Comb hair
  - Use a hammer
  - Turn a key.

Next, if there is difficulty in performing these acts to command, the patient is asked to imitate these movements when demonstrated by the examiner.

In examining for the presence of buccofacial apraxia, the patient is then asked to perform a series of facial movements to command. Again, if there is difficulty with these items, imitation is tested. These items might include asking the patient to demonstrate how they would:

- Blow out a candle
- Suck on a straw
- Cough
- Lick their lips.

Visuospatial and visuoconstructional functioning

Visuospatial functions involve the localization of objects or, indeed, the self in space. Visuoconstructional functioning, meanwhile, refers to the ability to form a whole object from an appreciation and manipulation of its constituent parts. Obviously, both these functions require vision to be intact and thus difficulties with visual perception should be considered before undertaking any of these measures.

Formal testing in this area offers a wide range of standardized instruments. However, it is still possible to use simpler tasks in situations that require some degree of screening evaluation but that are impractical or unsuitable to comprehensive testing.

Thus, visuospatial performance can be assessed by asking the patient to draw simple objects such as clock faces. Clock faces benefit from being simple, easily adapted, two-dimensional representations. Most patients will not, therefore, feel that the task demands a high degree of drawing skill and will not, as a result, feel intimidated. The examiner simply asks the patient to draw a clock face and to draw in the hands of the clock at a certain time (Fig. 11.2).

Interpretation of this measure will, of course, need to take into account any difficulties with visual acuity. However, certain types of error in drawing can highlight a number of different problems. For instance, the clock hands may not meet at a central point, the number arrangement may be incorrect, or the clock face itself could be asymmetrical. Another possibility is that if all of the numbers are confined to one side or the other of the clock face, this can suggest problems with visual neglect.

Visuospatial functioning, and particularly visual neglect phenomena, can also be tested by asking the patient to bisect lines of varying length into two equal parts. Patients demonstrating neglect consistently divide the line pro-

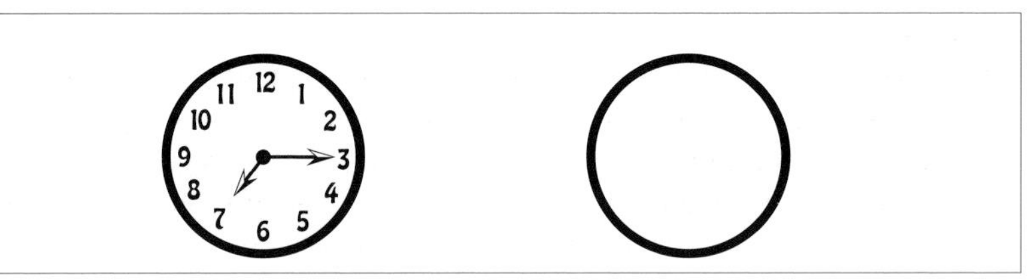

Fig. 11.2 A clock face – the patient is asked to draw or fill in the blank clock face with the hands set at, for example, 7:15.

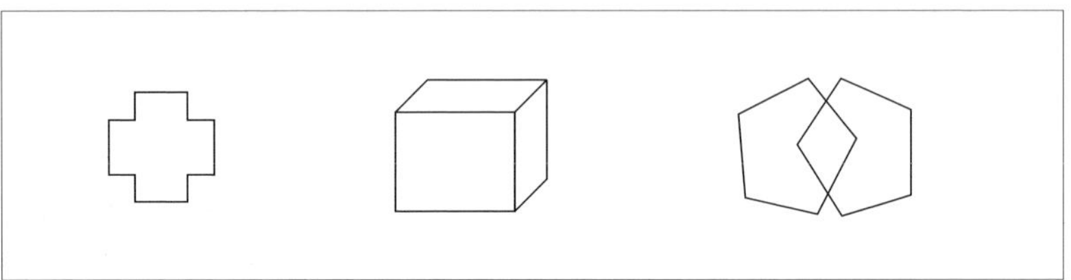

Fig. 11.3 Visuoconstruction – a cross, three-dimensional square and intersecting polygons.

vided beyond the mid-point and, as the line increases in length, so the patients will tend to demonstrate placement of the bisection marker further and further away from the mid-point.

Visuoconstructional functioning can be assessed both two and three-dimensionally. However, three-dimensional stimuli such as the coloured blocks provided on the Block Design sub-test of the WAIS-III are not commonly available. The testing of visuoconstructional abilities can, nevertheless, be achieved by asking the patient to copy simple two-dimensional and three-dimensional drawings such as those depicted in Figure 11.3.

Right-left orientation may also be assessed under the heading of spatial functioning, assessing the patient's personal space orientation and, to some degree, verbal comprehension. Naturally, some problems exist in the normal unaffected population and very often individuals can recount a history of 'not knowing their right from their left' and this, of course, should be taken into account. The examiner, therefore, suitably aware of the patient's history and handedness, and after excluding a language comprehension deficit, should give a series of increasingly complex verbal commands to the patient without demonstration. For example:

- Lift your right hand
- Lift your left hand
- Touch your left ear
- Touch your right ear
- Touch your right ear with your left hand
- Touch your left ear with your right hand
- Put your right hand on your left knee
- Put your left hand on your right knee.

SUMMARY

In this chapter, we have consolidated the learning from previous chapters and combined this with more practical tasks in order to give an introduction to basic assessment techniques. In so doing, we have examined factors related to the patient's background and presentation. These have included an appreciation of the medical history, features of the medical record and physical examination results.

We have also isolated a number of important factors that, quite apart from cerebral involvement, can also play a role in testing, such as mood state and level of cooperation. In addition, we have highlighted individual differences such as culture and educational background, which can also indirectly influence performance.

Finally, while accepting that screening assessment is not a replacement or substitute for professional neuropsychological assessment or specialist training, we have endeavoured to expand on the briefer testing methodologies and provide a foundation for understanding some of the essentials of basic cognitive assessment.

FURTHER READING

Armstrong M A 1997 The basic mental status examination series I: conducting the patient interview (video). Lippincott Williams and Wilkins, Philadelphia

Armstrong M A 1997 The basic mental status examination series II: evaluating aspects of appearance (video). Lippincott Williams and Wilkins, Philadelphia

Armstrong M A 1997 The basic mental status examination series III: evaluating language and thought patterns (video). Lippincott Williams and Wilkins, Philadelphia

Armstrong M A 1997 The basic mental status examination series IV: evaluating intellectual and cognitive function (video). Lippincott Williams and Wilkins, Philadelphia

Hodges J R 1994 Cognitive assessment for clinicians. Oxford Medical Publications, Oxford

Appendix I

There are numerous central nervous system (CNS) disorders. Equally, there are many medications that can be prescribed in order to deal with either the primary or secondary symptoms of these disorders and the other conditions that may arise as a consequence of CNS insult. In general, however, these medications do not cure or eradicate the presence of disorder. Rather, most medicines correct balances, block or enhance the action of certain neurotransmitter substances and modify cellular activity.

To attempt to describe the action and use of all of these drugs is, of course, beyond the scope of this book. Indeed, there are so many medications on the market and in development that such an undertaking would probably necessitate the writing of a second, companion volume. Moreover, as has already been made clear in Chapter 6 there are many pharmaceutical interventions which, although effective, are not necessarily associated with a specific condition. For example, antihypertensives may be used to treat high blood pressure and thus reduce the risk for stroke. These, however, are not directly associated with stroke treatment.

Instead, this short section will attempt to give a brief description of the application and effects of some of the major and more often encountered medications as they pertain to a limited number of specific disorders or secondary symptoms. It must be stressed, however, that what follows is by no means an exhaustive list of medications; nor is it intended to be a substitute for the much more comprehensive descriptions, indications and prescribing principles offered by other publications.

The reader is, therefore directed to the many fine texts available providing more thorough and detailed information, including:

Henry J A (ed) 2001 The British Medical Association new guide to medicines and drugs. Dorling Kindersley, London

Luker K, Wolfson D J 1998 Medicines management for clinical nurses. Blackwell Science (UK), Oxford

Dinesh M (ed) 2005 British National Formulary volume 49. Pharmaceutical Press, Oxon

The reader is also directed to the website for the British National Formulary which offers on-line access to the text on the selection, prescribing, dispensing and administration of medications, as well as to the latest update information.

http://bnf.org/bnf/

ANTICONVULSANTS

Anticonvulsant or antiepileptic drugs serve to reduce the risk and frequency of seizure through the reduction of the excitability of neuronal tissue, either by enhancing inhibitory processes or by suppressing stimulation. This is achieved by the maintenance of an optimal level of medication within the system, while at the same time striking a balance between control and side-effects.

However, because the nature of epilepsy is highly individual and the seizure threshold varies from person to person, there is no standard dose for anticonvulsants. Indeed, there will be occasions when a particular drug is not effective and several other medications are tried, or when a combination of drugs is needed to gain control.

Prior to prescription, then, an appraisal of the type of epilepsy suffered is required as this will govern the type of drug given. For example, valproate is effective in cases of primary generalized epilepsy, whereas phenytoin may be prescribed for partial seizures and carbamazepine for complex partial seizures. This is followed by monitoring and a careful increase in dosage until control is achieved.

In more difficult cases, where combination therapies (more than one medication) are given, there may also be a number of interactions that can occur between anticonvulsant medications, causing toxicity without necessarily improving seizure control. Monitoring in these cases, therefore, is even more important.

Anticonvulsant medications, by dint of their action, tend not only to control seizures but can produce unwanted side-effects. This is because the inhibitory process by which they act will also diminish normal brain function with potential secondary effects on cognition, etc. The type of side-effects that may be experienced will vary with the type of drug used but might generally be expected to include poor memory, poor concentration, poor coordination, fatigue, drowsiness, visual disturbance, dizziness and weight gain. Liver function may also be affected by anticonvulsant medication affecting the metabolism of other drugs. Many anticonvulsants also carry a risk in terms of fetal development during pregnancy.

Common drug names are shown in Box AI.1.

ANTIDEPRESSANTS

There are three main types of drug used to treat depression, each of which has a different action. These are the tricyclic antidepressants (TCAs), the selective serotonin re-uptake inhibitors (SSRIs) and the monoamine oxidase inhibitors (MAOIs).

TCAs act by blocking the re-uptake sites for the neurotransmitters serotonin and noradrenaline (norepinephrine) and, therefore, increasing the availability of these neurotransmitters. The SSRIs are a newer development and are generally considered to have fewer side-effects than the TCAs. They act to block the re-uptake of the neurotransmitter serotonin. The MAOIs, as

Box AI.1 Common anticonvulsant drug names

Approved name	Proprietary name
Carbamazepine	Tegretol
Clobazam	
Clonazepam	Rivotril
Ethosuximide	Zarontin
Gabapentin	Neurontin
Lamotrigine	Lamictal
Levetiracetam	Keppra
Oxcarbazepine	Trileptal
Phenobarbital	
Phenytoin	Epanutin
Primidone	Mysoline
Sodium valproate	Epilim
Tiagabine	Gabitril
Topiramate	Topamax
Vigabatrin	Sabril

their name implies, act by inhibiting the action of the enzyme responsible for the breakdown of monoamine neurotransmitters. Thus, this class of antidepressants increases the availability of serotonin, noradrenaline (norepinephrine) and dopamine. However, because of possible side-effects and potentially dangerous dietary interactions, MAOIs tend not to be the first choice for treatment.

The TCAs are useful when depression is associated with psychophysiological symptoms such as sleep disturbance or loss of appetite. Some TCAs are also used in the treatment of panic disorder, enuresis and neuropathic pain, and because of the sedating effect of some of these drugs, they can be helpful in the management of depression associated with anxiety and agitation. Side-effects include dry mouth, blurred vision, sweating, constipation, and urinary retention. TCAs are also associated with a reduction in seizure threshold and so should be used with caution in cases of epilepsy.

SSRIs, as previously stated, tend to have fewer side-effects than some of the TCAs. They also tend to be less sedating and are safer in cases of overdose. In general, however, this class of antidepressant is considered no more effective than the TCAs. Side-effects include nausea, vomiting, dry mouth, anxiety, headache, insomnia, dizziness and tremor. The SSRIs should also be used with caution in cases of epilepsy.

MAOIs are encountered far less frequently than either the TCAs or SSRIs. The reason for this is that, despite their efficacy, they can have dangerous interactions with items in the diet and with other drugs. To illustrate, MAOIs taken with foods rich in tyramine such as mature cheese, red wine, or yeast extracts can produce a dangerous increase in blood pressure. Patients taking these drugs, therefore, are provided with a list of prohibited food stuffs. Nevertheless, MAOIs can be effective in cases of atypical depression and phobic disorder.

It should also be noted that, although the above antidepressant can influence mood state, mood stabilizing effects are also noted with the use of the

Box AI.2 Common antidepressant drug names

Approved name	Proprietary name
TCAs	
Amitriptyline	
Chlomipramine	Anafranil
Dothiepin	Prothieden
Imipramine	Tofranil
Lofepramine	Gamanil
SSRIs	
Citalopram	Cipramil
Fluoxetine	Prozac
Paroxetine	Seroxat
Sertraline	Lustral
MAOIs	
Isocarboxazid	
Moclobemide	Manerix
Phenelzine	Nardil
Tranylcypromine	

anticonvulsant medications, carbamazepine and sodium valproate. Finally, it should also be noted that because of the potential for interaction and possible toxicity, the popular herbal remedy St John's wort should not be taken in conjunction with antidepressants.

Common drug names are shown in Box AI.2.

ANTIPSYCHOTICS

Antipsychotic or neuroleptic medication (sometimes referred to as major tranquillizers) can be used to treat psychotic symptoms in conditions such as schizophrenia. However, they can also be used to treat acute agitation in a number of other conditions such as brain damage and can also be used in the short term to treat severe anxiety.

In general, antipsychotics act by reducing the stimulation activity of the neurotransmitter dopamine with the brain. This is achieved by decreasing the level of activity in cells through a binding of dopamine antagonists to the receptor sites of cells, thus blocking the stimulatory effects of dopamine. Certain of the newer types of antipsychotic medication also serve to block receptor sites for the neurotransmitter serotonin.

Antipsychotic drugs can be categorized as typical and atypical, meaning that they either have the classical or typical antagonistic effect on dopamine, or that they have a lesser effect on dopamine activity but also affect other neurotransmitter activity such as serotonin, rendering them atypical.

As antipsychotics affect the actions of dopamine within the brain, they can produce a secondary imbalance in the neurotransmitter acetylcholine, causing a number of what are known as extrapyramidal side-effects. These

Box AI.3 Common antipsychotic drug names

Approved name	Proprietary name
Typical antipsychotics	
Benperidol	Benquil
Chlopromazine hydrochloride	Largactil
Flupenthixol	Depixol
Fluphenazine hydrochloride	Modecate, Moditen
Haloperidol	Haldol, Serenance, Dozic
Levomepromazine	Nozinan
Pericyazine	Neulactil
Pimozide	Orap
Promazine hydrochloride	
Sulparide	Dolmatil, Sulpitil, Sulpor
Thioridazine	Melleril
Tripfluoperazine	Stelazine
Zuclopenthixol acetate	Clopixol, Acuphase
Zuclopenthixol dihydrochloride	Clopixol
Atypical antipsychotics	
Amisulpride	Solian
Clozapine	Clozaril
Olanzepine	Zyprexa
Quetiapine	Seroquel
Risperidone	Risperdal
Sertindole	Serodelect
Zotepine	Zoleptil

are side-effects involving the extrapyramidal structures of the brain, a collection of cortical and subcortical structures involved in motor functions.

These side-effects can include tremor, dystonia, tardive dyskinesia, and akathesia, as well as hypotension and problems with temperature regulation. Other side-effects can include dizziness, blurred vision, dry mouth, tachycardia, drowsiness, agitation, confusion, gastrointestinal disturbance, constipation, sleep disturbance, changes in menstruation, impotence and weight gain.

It should also be noted that some of these agents can interact with anticonvulsant medication, lowering seizure threshold. Also, a potentially lethal side-effect of antipsychotic use is a condition known as neuroleptic malignant syndrome (NMS). This is characterized by tachycardia, difficulties with blood pressure, muscular rigidity, urinary incontinence, sweating, hyperthermia and fluctuating levels of consciousness. However, it should be stressed that this is not a frequent occurrence with antipsychotic use.

Common drug names are shown in Box AI.3.

ANXIOLYTICS

Anxiolytics or anti-anxiety drugs are prescribed in order to ease persistent problems with tension, agitation and nervousness. Many will also provide a

Box AI.4 Common anxiolytic drug names

Approved name	Proprietary name
Benzodiazepines	
Alprazolam	Xanax
Chlordiazepoxide	
Diazepam	
Oxazepam	
Lorazepam	
Beta-blockers	
Atenolol	Tenormin
Propranolol	Inderal

sedative property, aiding sleep at night. Similarly, many hypnotics, prescribed to aid difficulties with persistent sleeplessness problems, will provide a sedating effect during the day. Broadly, there are two types of anti-anxiety drug: benzodiazepines and beta-blockers, each of which has different effects.

Benzodiazepines act upon the psychological symptoms of anxiety by enhancing the inhibitory effects of the neurotransmitter gamma-amminobutyric acid (GABA) and are the most commonly used anxiolytic, being prescribed for all manner of minor and major anxiety states. However, although these drugs are effective, there is also a likelihood of dependence and tolerance. Their use, therefore, is usually limited to as low a dose as possible over a short period of time. In addition, like most medicines, benzodiazepines do not resolve the causes of anxiety but merely treat the symptoms. Psychological therapies, therefore, offer the best solution for long-term resolution and, indeed, in certain cases, can actually delay psychological adjustment. Side-effects include drowsiness, dizziness, forgetfulness, and dependence.

Beta-blockers, on the other hand, are used mainly to reduce the physical symptoms of anxiety and do not directly affect psychological symptoms. Thus, they are regularly prescribed in order to reduce physical symptoms occurring in specific situations such as the anxiety caused by public speaking, interviews or examinations. This class of drugs acts by blocking the action of adrenaline and noradrenaline (epinephrine and norepinephrine) and reducing the physical symptoms of anxiety such as raised heart rate. Side-effects can include bradycardia, hypotension, respiratory difficulties, fatigue and sleep disturbance.

Common drug names are shown in Box AI.4.

DRUGS USED TO TREAT ALZHEIMER'S DISEASE

The cognitive decline associated with Alzheimer's disease (AD) is thought to be related to the cholinergic pathways of a number of subcortical structures and their projections to the cortex. In AD, then, drugs that enhance cholinergic function are prescribed. Thus, drugs that inhibit the action of the enzyme acetylcholinesterase, which breaks down the neurotransmitter acetylcholine, are used to treat mild to moderate forms.

Box AI.5 Names of common drugs used to treat Alzheimer's disease

Approved name	Proprietary name
Donepezil hydrochloride	Aricept
Galantamine	Reminyl
Rivastigmine	Exelon

The use of these medications is closely linked to repeated cognitive assessment and evaluation of the patient's response to treatment, with evidence suggesting that a large proportion of cases will demonstrate a slower rate of decline. In most uncomplicated cases, initial assessment and monitoring is achieved using the Mini-Mental Status Examination (MMSE).

Acetylcholinesterase inhibitors, however, can cause a number of dose-related side-effects associated with cholinergic functions. Like anticonvulsant medication, therefore, the dose of medication must be carefully increased in order to strike a balance between side-effects and cognitive enhancement. Such side-effects can include nausea, vomiting, diarrhoea, weight loss, fatigue, dizziness, headache and confusion.

Common drug names are shown in Box AI.5.

DRUGS USED TO TREAT PARKINSON'S DISEASE AND PARKINSONISM

These drugs broadly fall into two categories: dopaminergic medications used to enhance or increase the levels of available dopamine and antimuscarinic medications used to reduce the levels of cholinergic function that can increase as a result of dopamine deficiency.

Dopamine levels within the brain cannot be increased directly. The substance is poorly absorbed in the digestive tract and does not cross the blood–brain barrier. Therefore, treatment is effected by either giving dopamine in a form which can be utilized by the body and converted; by reducing the breakdown of naturally occurring dopamine; by a prolongation of the action of naturally occurring dopamine within the brain; or by a combination of these treatments.

Treatment with dopaminergics does not usually commence until symptoms begin to cause considerable difficulties with daily activities. This is partly because many of these agents have a fixed span of use and, although they can help to manage symptoms, they do not cure the underlying cause of the disorder. Thus, while these medications may be used for many years, they can gradually demonstrate a decreased effect on symptoms while at the same time producing an increasing level of side-effects. Dosage and frequency may, therefore, have to be increased.

The choice of medication or combination of medications is governed by the individual case, the symptoms presented, the degree to which the symptoms are exhibited, and the potential for side-effects. The side-effects of the dopaminergic medications can vary a great deal and can include weight loss, nausea, vomiting, postural hypotension, dizziness, tachycardia, sleep disturbance, dyskinesia, mood disturbances, cognitive impairment and psychotic phenomena, particularly in prolonged use.

Antimuscarinic medications, on the other hand, restore chemical balance by reducing increased acetylcholine activity within the brain caused by a reduction in the levels of dopamine. This class of drugs is effective in cases of drug-induced Parkinsonism; for example Parkinsonism caused by the use of antipsychotic drugs which decrease levels of dopamine. However, antimuscarinic drugs are generally less effective in cases of idiopathic Parkinson's disease (PD) and, although they can help to reduce tremor and rigidity, they have almost no impact on bradykinesia.

The side-effects of this class of medication can produce a wide range of anticholinergic signs. These can include sedation, cognitive impairment, dry mouth, gastrointestinal upset, blurred vision, dizziness, tachycardia, agitation, insomnia, and in some cases, psychiatric disturbances at higher doses.

Common drug names are shown in Box AI.6.

Box AI.6 Names of common drugs used to treat Parkinson's disease and Parkinsonism

Approved name	Proprietary name
Dopaminergics	
Amatadine hydrochloride	Symmetrel
Apomorphine hydrochloride	APO-Go
Bromocriptine	
Cabergoline	Cabaser
Co-beneldopa	Madopar
Co-careldopa	Sinemet
Entacopone	Comtess
Levodopa	
Lisuride	Maleate
Pergolide	Celance
Pramipexole	Mirapexin
Ropinorole	Requip
Selegiline hydrochloride	Eldepryl, Zelapar
Antimuscarinics	
Benzatropine mesilate	Cogentin
Biferiden hydrochloride	Akineton
Orphenadrine hydrochloride	Biorphen, Disipal
Procyclidine hydrochloride	Kemadrin, Arpicolin
Trihexphenidyl hydrochloride	Broflex

Appendix II

Below is a list of various internet website addresses for those seeking further information. This list is broken down into a number of subsections that includes professional bodies and scientific societies, neuropsychology and neurology resources, support groups, journals and neuropsychological test publishers and resource companies.

SOCIETIES

American Academy of Neurology (ANN)
http://www.aan.com/professionals/
American Neurological Association (ANA)
http://www.aneuroa.org/
American Neuropsychiatric Association (ANPA)
http://www.anpaonline.org/
American Psychological Association (APA)
http://www.apa.org/
http://www.div40.org/
Association of British Neurologists (ABN)
http://www.theabn.org/
British Association for Psychopharmacology (BAP)
http://www.bap.org.uk/
British Neuropsychiatry Association (BNPA)
http://www.bnpa.org.uk/
British Neuropsychological Society (BNS)
http://www.psychology.nottingham.ac.uk/bns/
British Psychological Society (BPS)
http://www.bps.org.uk/index.cfm
International Neuropsychology Society (INS)
http://www.the-ins.org/
National Academy of Neuropsychology (NAN)
http://nanonline.org/
Society for Neuroscience (SFN)
http://web.sfn.org/
World Federation for Neurology (WFN)
http://www.wfneurology.org/

NEUROPSYCHOLOGY AND NEUROLOGY RESOURCES

The internet offers a wealth of information on neuropsychological and neurological disorders, some of it good and some of it not so good. Below, then, are listed just a few of the more useful and interesting sites available.

BrainInfo

A site designed to provide identification and information on brain structures.
http://braininfo.rprc.washington.edu/

The Institute of Neurology

The website of the Institute of Neurology in Queens Square, London, offering information on various conditions, research links and other neuroscience resources.
http://www.ion.ucl.ac.uk/

The Institute of Psychiatry

The website of the Institute of Psychiatry in London. The site offers a variety of mental health information and has a neuroscience page providing information on disorders and links to other resources.
http://www.iop.kcl.ac.uk/

Medicine Guides

An information source intended for members of the public, offering information on certain medicines and links to various other pharmacological sites and professional pharmacological bodies.
http://www.medicines.org.uk/

Neuroguide

A searchable database of web based neuroscience resources.
http://www.neuroguide.com/

Neuropsychology Central

Certainly the best dedicated neuropsychological website, containing a variety of information on neuropsychology and presenting links to other resources including organizations, training in the USA, treatment and software.
http://www.neuropsychologycentral.com/

Net Doctor

A searchable database of medical information, examinations, treatments, medicines, discussions and support.
http://www.netdoctor.co.uk/

NHS Direct

The National Health Service portal offering links to conditions, treatments and local services directories, etc.
http://www.nhsdirect.nhs.uk/

Psych-Net (UK)

Dedicated to psychological sciences and mental health issues, this site offers links to terminology, research, articles, discussion forums, and software, etc., as well as having specific pages devoted to neuroscience and neuropsychology.
http://www.psychnet-uk.com/

The Whole Brain Atlas

A collection of useful and informative atlas of neuroanatomy images with additional neuropathological MRI, CT, PET and SPECT studies.
http://www.med.harvard.edu/AANLIB/home.html

SUPPORT GROUPS

There are many groups locally, nationally and internationally that help to support the needs of sufferers. Below is a list of the main support groups in the UK.

Dementia

The Alzheimer's Research Trust
Website: http://www.alzheimers-research.org.uk/
Email: enquiries@alzheimers-research.org.uk
The Alzheimer's Society
Website: http://www.alzheimers.org.uk/
Email: enquiries@alzheimers.org.uk

Epilepsy

The National Society for Epilepsy
Website: http://www.epilepsynse.org.uk/
Epilepsy Action (The British Epilepsy Association)
Website: http://epilepsy.org.uk/

Head injury

Headway
Website: http://www.headway.org.uk/
Email: information@headway.org.uk

Multiple sclerosis

The Multiple Sclerosis Society
Website: http://www.mssociety.org.uk/
Email: info@mssociety.org.uk
The Multiple Sclerosis Trust
Website: http://www.msresearchtrust.org.uk
Email: info@mstrust.org.uk

Parkinson's disease

The Parkinson's Disease Society
Website: http://www.parkinsons.org.uk/
Email: enquiries@parkinsons.org.uk
Young Alert Parkinson's and Relatives
Website: http://www.youngonset-parkinsons.org.uk/
Email: webmaster@yap-web.org.uk

Stroke (CVA)

The Stroke Association
Website: http://www.stroke.org.uk/
Email: info@stroke.org.uk

Other

The Encephalitis Society
Website: http://www.encephalitis.info/Home.asp
Email: mail@encephalitis.info
The Huntington's Disease Association
Website: http://www.hda.org.uk/
Email: info@hda.org.uk
Meningitis Trust
Website: http://www.meningitis-trust.org/
Email: info@meningitis-trust.org
Migraine Action Association
Website: http://www.migraine.org.uk/
Email: info@migraine.org.uk
Motor Neurone Disease Action
Website: http://www.mndassociation.org/full-site/home.shtml
Email: enquiries@mndassociation.org
Tourette's Syndrome (UK) Association
Website: http://www.tsa.org.uk/
Email: enquiries@tsa.org.uk

JOURNALS

The list of available journals is extensive. I have, therefore, detailed below a number of the more popular and relevant publications. This list is broken down first into journals that can be accessed on-line and, second, journals that can be ordered on-line.

Journals with on-line access

Archives of Neurology
http://archneur.ama-assn.org/
Brain
http://brain.oxfordjournals.org/
British Medical Journal
http://bmj.bmjjournals.com/
Cortex
http://www.cortex-online.org/
Journal of Neurology, Neurosurgery and Psychiatry
http://jnnp.bmjjournals.com/
Journal of Neuropsychiatry
http://intl-neuro.psychiatryonline.org/
The Lancet
http://www.thelancet.com/
Neurology
http://www.neurology.org/
New England Journal of Medicine
http://content.nejm.org/
Stroke
http://intl-stroke.ahajournals.org/

Journals available for on-line ordering

Annals of Neurology
http://www3.interscience.wiley.com/cgi-bin/jhome/76507645
The Clinical Neuropsychologist
http://www.tandf.co.uk/journals/titles/13854046.asp
Cognitive Neuropsychology
http://www.tandf.co.uk/journals/titles/02643294.asp
Journal of Clinical and Experimental Neuropsychology
http://www.tandf.co.uk/journals/titles/13803395.asp
Journal of the International Neuropsychology Society
http://www.cambridge.org/uk/journals/journal_catalogue.asp?mnemonic=ins
Laterality
http://www.tandf.co.uk/journals/titles/1357650x.asp
Neurocase
http://www.tandf.co.uk/journals/titles/13554794.asp

NEUROPSYCHOLOGICAL TEST PUBLISHERS AND RESOURCE COMPANIES

For those interested in looking in more detail at the tests described in Chapter 10, I have listed below some of the main test suppliers along with the acronyms of some of the measures discussed in the main body of the preceding text.

Harcourt Assessment

Incorporating the Psychological Corporation and the Thames Valley Test Company, this publisher now markets the WAIS-III, WMS-III, WMS-III A, KBNA, RBANS, BDI-II, and BAI, etc.
Website: http://www.harcourt-uk.com/

Nfer-Nelson

Providing a range of instruments, Nfer-Nelson also publishes a number of items for use in health and social care settings. Amongst these are the HADS.
Website: http://www.nfer-nelson.co.uk/

Pearson Assessments

Formerly NCS Assessments, this company produces a range of neuropsychological instruments and also supplies the MMPI-2.
Website: http://www.pearsonassessments.com/

Psychological Assessment Resources (PAR)

Marketing a wide-range of testing resources, psychometric instruments, books and software, PAR retails items such as SNST, SCWT, JLO, WCST and TOMM.
Website: http://www3.parinc.com/

The Reitan Neuropsychology Laboratory

Supplying the HRB, this company produces all of the items needed to administer this comprehensive battery.
Website: http://www.reitanlabs.com/

Western Psychological Services (WPS)

WPS supplies a number of assessments, books, software, and tools for use by psychologists. This company also provides the LNNB.
Website: http://www.wpspublish.com/Inetpub4/index.htm

Glossary

Acalculia – An inability to perform mathematical computations.

Affect – The emotional state of an individual at any given time.

Agnosia – An inability to recognize objects or forms. Occurring after damage to the brain, it can be manifest in any sensory modality despite intact perception and memory.

Agraphia – An acquired disorder of writing skills.

Akathesia – Restlessness, an urge for movement.

Alexia – An acquired reading disorder.

Amnesia – A total or partial loss of memory.

Anaesthesia – A partial or complete loss of sensitivity.

Anarithmetria – Inability to perform mathematical computations: to add, subtract, multiply or divide. It is often disturbed in reverse order, i.e. division is first to be affected and addition last.

Aneurysm – The dilation of the wall of an artery.

Angiography – A visualization of blood vessels of the arterial system after the injection of an opaque contrast medium.

Anomia – Inability to name objects. It is a symptom of aphasia.

Anorgasmia – Inability to achieve orgasm.

Anterograde – Progressing forward in time. It is often applied to amnesia and indicates loss of recall of information following an event. It is the opposite of retrograde.

Aphasia – A set of language disorders resulting from damage to the brain. It is also called dysphasia.

Apraxia – An inability to perform skilful or purposeful movement despite a lack of paralysis or sensory disturbance.

Ataxia – The partial or complete loss of motor coordination.

Bilateral – Pertaining to both sides of a given space or, in this case, the brain.

Central nervous system – That part of the nervous system consisting of the brain and spinal cord. It is often abbreviated to CNS.

Cerebral – Pertaining to the cerebrum.

Cerebral dominance – The proposal that one hemisphere of the brain is dominant to the other in terms of function. This is observed in the dominance of one hemisphere for speech and movement. Frequently, the terms hemispheric specialization and laterality are used in place of cerebral dominance.

Cerebral spinal fluid – Similar to blood plasma, this fluid bathes and supports the brain and spinal cord, acting as a transport medium for nutrients to the neurons. It is also referred to as cerebrospinal fluid and abbreviated as CSF.

Cerebrovascular event – A disturbance of the cerebral blood flow due to haemorrhage, embolism or thrombosis. The term is interchangeable with cerebrovascular accident (CVA) and is often abbreviated to CVE.

Cerebrum – Responsible for higher functioning, the cerebrum is the largest and most prominent feature of the brain; it consists of two hemispheres divided by the longitudinal fissure. The inner core is composed of white matter and is surrounded by a thinner outer layer, the cerebral cortex, which is composed of grey matter cells.

Closed head injury – Damage to the brain sustained as a result of the forceful impact of the head with another object but without penetration of the brain. It is often abbreviated as CHI.

Cognition – A broad term taken to refer to mental activities such as thought, memory, problem-solving, etc.

Confabulation – The filling in of gaps in memory with fabricated information.

Contralateral – Pertaining to the opposite side; for example a cerebrovascular accident involving the left cerebral hemisphere might result in a right-sided or contralateral weakness.

CT scan – A series of computerized X-rays taken at different levels of the brain.

Demyelination – A destruction of the myelin sheath surrounding nerve fibres.

Diplopia – Double vision.

Dysdiadochokinesia – Difficulty in performing rapid alternating movements. It is often observed as difficulties between the fingers or hands on either side of the body; its presence is an instance of a soft neurological sign, a subtle indicator of possible brain damage. When alternating rapid movements cannot be performed this sign is called adiadochokinesia.

Dysmetria – A difficulty with the assessment and accomplishment of the range and force of movement. It is often observed as the over or undershooting of movement towards a target; for example problems with the picking up of a cup caused by reaching too far or too close for it.

Dysphagia – Difficulty with swallowing.

Dysphoria – A disturbance of mood often caused by anxiety or depression.

Dystonia – An impairment of muscle tone.

Echolalia – The repetition of words or phrases.

Electroencephalogram (EEG) – a recording of the brain's electrical activity.

Emotional lability – A tendency to abrupt, unpredictable and inappropriate emotional changes.

Fasiculation – An involuntary twitching of muscle groups.

Foramen – An opening or passageway. It is generally used to refer to openings in bones; for example the foramen magnum is the opening in the occipital bone of the skull through which the spinal cord passes.

Foramina – The plural of foramen.
Hemiplegia – Paralysis involving one half of the body.
Hypergraphia – Excessive writing activity.
Hyperphonia – Excessively loud in volume.
Hypersomnolence – Excessive sleepiness.
Ideation – Pertaining to ideas, thoughts or cognitive processes.
Infarction – Premature and irreversible death of the tissues.
Intrathecal – a term meaning 'within the meninges'. It is often used to refer to a medication route between the meninges of the spinal cord.
Ischaemia – A deficient blood supply. For example, a transient ischaemic attack (TIA) involves the brief interruption of the blood supply to an area of the brain.
Kinaesthesis – A sense of movement; a muscle sense.
Lateralization – The process by which different functions are associated with one side of the brain or the other. For example, in most individuals, the bulk of language function is lateralized to the left hemisphere of the brain.
Lesion – A pathological change in tissue. For example, an MRI scan may demonstrate a lesion or a circumscribed area or damage to a particular area of the brain.
Localization – Also known as the localization of function, this term pertains to the location of specific functions within specific structures or areas of the brain.
Mnesis – Memory.
MRI scan – The use of magnetic fields to produce images of the brain that provide more detailed images than CT scans.
Neuralgia – Pain experienced along the pathway of a nerve.
Nystagmus – Jerky, repetitive movements of the eye.
Ophthalmoplegia – A paralysis of one or more of the eye muscles resulting in difficulties with incorrect eye movement.
Pathogenesis – The origin and development of illness.
Paraesthesia – An abnormality of sensation, for example persistent tingling sensations.
Paresis – A partial paralysis leading to weakness.
Paroxysm – A fit, convulsion or attack.
Paroxysmal – Something which occurs as attacks or in paroxysms. For example, epileptic seizures are paroxysmal in nature.
Penetrating head injury – Damage to the brain sustained as a result of the penetration of the skull by an object such as a missile. It is often abbreviated as PHI.
Perseveration – A tendency to inappropriately continue or exhibit ideational or behavioural action.
Phagocyte – A cell capable of engulfing and digesting other particles such as bacteria.
Physiogenesis – Developing from physical origins.
Plegia – Used in conjunction with a number of prefixes to signify paralysis; for example hemiplegia means on one side of the body and paraplegia refers to paralysis in the lower limbs.

Prodromal – Referring to the earliest stages of a disorder or illness and pertaining to the appearance of the first symptom but before the manifestation of the disorder.

Proprioception – The perception of body parts and their movement.

Prosody – The sound pattern of a speech utterance. For example, a rising inflection at the end of an interrogative sentence denotes a question and is, therefore, part of the prosodic components of that utterance.

Psychogenesis – Developing from psychological origins.

Retrograde – Progressing backward in time. Often applied to amnesia and indicating loss of recall for information before an event. It is the opposite of anterograde.

Schema – A cognitive model representing personal knowledge regarding the arrangement of body parts and their spatial relationship to objects in the environment.

Simultagnosia – Difficulties in the perception of different aspects of the same object or a scene in the visual field. Sufferers, therefore, are able to perceive individual features of the object or scene but are unable to recognize the whole.

Somnolence – Sleepiness or drowsiness.

Spasticity – An abnormal increase in muscle tone.

Tardive dyskinesia – A disorder of involuntary movement involving the face and upper body, which usually involves lip-smacking, tongue protrusion, chewing movements, etc. It is a side-effect of many antipsychotic drugs.

Topographical disorientation – A type of visuospatial disorder leading to errors in spatial mapping and problems, with the result that sufferers are not able to navigate in familiar environments.

Trephination – The procedure of boring a hole in the skull.

Uhthoff's sign – A temporary blurring of vision related to an increase in body temperature. It is associated with multiple sclerosis and the sign can be elicited by a hot bath, exercise, and even emotional stress. Also known as Uhthoff's syndrome and Uhthoff's phenomenon.

Unilateral – Pertaining to one side of space or, this case, the brain.

Ventricle – A small cavity. For example, in the brain there are four ventricles filled with cerebral spinal fluid; in the heart there are two chambers called ventricles.

Ventricles – The four cavities of the brain filled with cerebrospinal fluid.

Visuoconstructive ability – Refers to the perceptual skill of copying or reproducing visually presented stimuli, two-dimensional drawings or three-dimensional blocks, etc.

Visuospatial – The ability to successfully deal with the spatial relationships between stimuli presented visually. Disturbance of this ability results in difficulty localizing objects in two- and three-dimensional space.

Visuoperceptive – The ability to perceive stimuli visually.

INDEX

Note: page numbers in **bold** refer to figures or boxes.

A

B

C

D

M

N

O

P

Q

R

S

T

U

V